Bipolar and Pregnant

Bipolar and Pregnant

How to Manage and Succeed in Planning and Parenting While Living with Manic Depression

Kristin K. Finn

Health Communications, Inc.
Deerfield Beach, Florida

www.hcibooks.com

Extracts on pages 3–4 and page 126 reprinted by permission of National Alliance on Mental Illness (NAMI).

Extracts on pages 8, 64, and 68–69 reprinted by permission of Guilford Publications, Inc.

Extract on page 22 reprinted by permission of www.realsavvymoms.com, Copyright 2007.

Extracts on pages 22–24, 25–26 and pages 79–81 reprinted by permission of March of Dimes.

Extracts on pages 34–37 reprinted by permission of Mental Health America.

Extract on pages 157–159 reprinted by permission of BabyCenter.

Extracts on pages 177–180 reprinted by permission of Depression and Bipolar Support Alliance (DBSA).

Extract on pages 182–183 reprinted by permission of Postpartum Support International (PSI).

Library of Congress Cataloging-in-Publication Data

Finn, Kristin K.
    Bipolar and pregnant : how to manage and succeed in planning and parenting while living with manic depression / Kristin K. Finn.
      p. cm.
    Includes bibliographical references and index.
    ISBN-13: 978-0-7573-0683-9 (trade paper : alk. paper)
    ISBN-10: 0-7573-0683-7 (trade paper : alk. paper)
    1. Finn, Kristin K.—Mental health. 2. Manic-depressive persons—United States—Biography. 3. Pregnant women—United States—Biography. 4. Pregnancy in mentally ill women. I. Title.

RC516.F47 2007
616.89'50092—dc22
[B]   2007021548

Publisher: Health Communications, Inc.
        3201 S.W. 15th Street
        Deerfield Beach, FL 33442-8190

Cover photo ©Corbis
Cover design by Larissa Hise Henoch
Interior design and formatting by Lawna Patterson Oldfield

Contents

Acknowledgments

I want to thank my incredibly supportive and patient husband, Fred, and my daughters, Katherine and Holly, who adapted their lives to make this book possible. I love them with all my heart. Katherine also helped to fine-tune the manuscript in its final stages, and Holly was always there to make me laugh when I needed to lighten up.

Thank you, Jay Carter, for encouraging me to write this book, for helping me to structure its contents, and for your feedback.

A special thanks to my contributors: Jay Carter, Ingrid Eerdmans, Fred Finn, Judith Hiemenga, Marjorie McCulloch, and Helga Valdmanis Toriello. Their perspectives were invaluable.

Rebecca Austin, my dear friend, thank you for believing in me and for your work in developing the manuscript. Your ongoing encouragement brightened my days.

A heartfelt thanks to my mother, Marjorie McCulloch, for helping me to edit the manuscript from start to finish.

I am also grateful for the feedback and encouragement I received from my father, David McCulloch; my brothers, Andrew and Michael McCulloch; Ginger Williams; Karen Mirque, P.T.;

Pauline A. Zazula, R.N.C.; Andrew MacDowell, M.D.; Carolyn MacDowell, R.N.; Nancy Roberts, R.N.; and Ruth Rupp Ryan.

Mary Jo Zazueta, thank you for professionally copyediting the first draft of the manuscript. Judith Antonelli, thank you for copyediting the final draft.

Robert West, my literary agent, gave me vision, support, and direction.

Finally, thanks to Michele Matrisciani, my editor at Health Communications, Inc., for her confidence in my work and for emphasizing the importance of this book for people affected with bipolar disorder and practitioners in the mental health community.

Preface

In April 1979, when I was almost seventeen, I was diagnosed with bipolar disorder* and began taking lithium. In September 1989, I married my husband, Fred, and in October 1990 we wanted to start a family. There is a degree of uncertainty in any pregnancy. We knew there would be additional challenges because of my bipolar disorder. There would possibly be medication adjustments and lifestyle changes. Our primary goals were to have a healthy baby and to manage my bipolar disorder both before and during the pregnancy.

Fred and I met with a genetic counselor, who reviewed our family histories and the risks that lithium and the other medications I was taking could create for the baby. Initially, after this meeting, we were discouraged—then we felt empowered and determined. We felt discouraged because she pointed out the genetic risks. It scared us, and self-doubt temporarily took over. Fred and I talked about our fears and knew we were ready to face them. We believed that we could work as a team to handle future challenges one step at a time.

---

*The terms *bipolar disorder, bipolar condition, bipolar,* and *chemical imbalance* are used interchangeably throughout the book. An expanded definition of *chemical imbalance* includes the way a person's brain uses and processes chemicals as well as external influences.

Bipolar and Pregnant describes my personal experiences, challenges, and coping methods through two pregnancies. It is the first book to share techniques and insights, from preconception through postpartum, written by a bipolar woman. This information is not just for the bipolar woman planning to have a child, however, but also for her entire support team and support network, which include individuals who provide any type of encouragement, medical care, and emotional support.

All pregnant women need support before, during, and after those nine months. Such support is even more important for a bipolar woman, who might think that standard pregnancy books and personal advice are not adequate to help with her unique needs. Bipolar disorder can be challenging to manage, but this book addresses these challenges and gives hope and guidance.

My passion is to help others with bipolar disorder plan and manage a pregnancy. When I first decided to write this book, I didn't know where to begin, so I talked with a friend in the publishing business. She suggested that I visit bookstores and the library to research other books on the subject. I discovered that very little has been written on this important topic, and I was immediately encouraged.

I then spoke with Ingrid Eerdmans, M.D., the psychiatrist who monitors my medication. I shared with her my intense interest in learning more about bipolar disorder and writing a book. Dr. Eerdmans suggested that I postpone writing because of my time commitments to my two daughters, my husband, and my career. Although I agreed, I felt both relieved and disappointed.

I chose not to dwell on it, believing that someday the timing would be right.

Continuing my journey in bipolar education, I attended a seminar about a year later on bipolar disorder for medical professionals, developed and presented by Jay Carter, PsyD, DABPS. I was one of the few nonprofessional attendees. At the beginning of his seminar, Dr. Carter stated that there is little practical information and advice on bipolar disorder and pregnancy from someone who has been there. He encouraged the audience to share what they thought would be valuable to the rest of the group.

Dr. Carter's invitation reinforced my decision to talk with him both during a break and after the seminar. I summarized my history and told him how I had managed both of my pregnancies, relying in part on the guidance of a pregnancy journal I maintained. He stated emphatically, "You should write a book. It could help a lot of people." The timing was right!

Some bipolars might not know many people who are familiar with their condition or who can relate to it. They might not have a supportive family or access to medical care for their chemical imbalance. To plan or even dream about having a baby can conjure up feelings of fear and despair if you have little or no guidance.

I hope that the details of my experiences, along with the expert knowledge from the contributors, will help you to feel empowered, hopeful, and ready to take the steps toward a healthy and enjoyable motherhood.

In order to provide the most accurate and valuable information about genetics, obstetrics, and medications as they relate to bipolar disorder, I have enlisted the advice of the following experts in the field:

Jay Carter, PsyD, DABPS, Fellow Prescribing Psychologist Register (FPPR) candidate, licensed psychologist, bestselling author, and lecturer, discusses executive functions in the brain in the course of the bipolar process, the importance of sleep and maintaining a routine as keys to avoiding bipolar episodes, and his relevant experience growing up with an untreated bipolar mother.

Ingrid Eerdmans, M.D., adult and child psychiatrist with twenty-five years of clinical experience, offers insights on postpartum disorders.

Judith Hiemenga, M.D., ob-gyn, concentrates on the medical aspects of pregnancy, preparing for pregnancy, and optimizing the chances of getting pregnant while decreasing the risks of psychiatric flare-ups.

Helga Valdmanis Toriello, Ph.D., Fellow of the American College of Medical Genetics (FACMG), medical geneticist, and director of Spectrum Health Genetics, writes about genetic counseling, the current research on medications used to treat bipolar disorder, and their effects on developing babies.

Fred Finn, my husband, shares his perspective and coping skills for partners and family members throughout this book. His insights as a supporter and new father are practical and heartfelt.

Marjorie McCulloch, R.N., my mother, provides reflections from the perspective of a former labor and delivery nurse, a health educator for the March of Dimes, a Michigan Genetics Advisory Board member, a prenatal class instructor, and, of course, a mother.

My husband, family, physicians, and friends helped me to conquer the unique challenges that my pregnancies brought. This book will show you, step by step, how to plan, manage, and cope with each phase of your pregnancy. I am privileged to share my experience with you.

Introduction

INGRID EERDMANS, M.D.

A planned pregnancy requires many considerations. The couple will review their financial situation to assess their ability to cover medical costs, the short-term and possibly long-term loss of a spouse's wages, and the cost of raising a child. They will assess their housing situation for a need to expand or move to accommodate their growing family. Individually and as a couple, they will determine if they are emotionally and psychologically prepared for the increased responsibility and curtailed freedom that a baby brings. They will consider their available support options, including the strength of their marriage and plans for child care. Perhaps most important, they will take into account the mother's health. Preexisting conditions, such as diabetes or multiple prior miscarriages indicate a high-risk pregnancy. I would include bipolar disorder among the conditions for which careful planning is necessary in order to lessen the risk as much as possible.

Unfortunately, although numbers and statistics about bipolar disorder in pregnancy are informative, they are too easily prone to distortion. For instance, postpartum psychosis (which is also called postpartum depression) is considered a medical emergency, for although it normally occurs in only 1–4 of every 1,000 women, it occurs in 50 percent of all postpartum women who have been diagnosed with bipolar disorder. Nevertheless, some bipolar women will hear this and think, "Yes, that's what happens to other people, but it would never happen to me," and they bury their heads in the sand. Other bipolar women will think that this consequence is inevitable and believe that their postpartum time is doomed. The previous mind-sets illustrate opposite ends of the spectrum, whereas Kristin's message is middle ground. There likely will be difficulties, but they can be managed.

That's why Kristin Finn's personal account of her journey through pregnancy and the postpartum period is so useful. She provides a real-life story that lends perspective to the numbers. Her coping strategies are practical, helpful, and easily implemented. Most important, her experience offers hope in its basic message: the obstacles that challenge women affected with bipolar disorder can be overcome, and a positive outcome can be realized.

Chapter 1

Getting Started: Looking at the Risks

F red and I understood the importance of reviewing the facts before making a decision to start a family. Was parenthood worth the risks involved in managing my own moods without medication, let alone potential risks to our baby? The questions in our minds were spiraling endlessly. We needed answers.

In October 1990, Fred and I had an appointment for genetic counseling at Spectrum Health Genetics in Grand Rapids, Michigan. Judy Hiemenga, M.D., my obstetrician-gynecologist, referred us. Our primary concern was what might happen to our baby if I continued to take lithium while pregnant. We also wanted to learn about the potential risks of continuing any of the prescriptions or over-the-counter drugs I was taking. My mother joined us at this meeting to provide moral support and to help in the review of our family history.

Scheduling an appointment with a genetic counselor before conception is a wise first step in planning any pregnancy, especially if you're affected with bipolar disorder. Asking your ob-gyn to refer you to a genetic counselor works well because the doctor is familiar with your history and can easily send your records. I encourage you to bring a family member who is familiar with your health history—and if that's not possible, then bring as much pertinent information with you as you can.

Because I was taking lithium (lithium carbonate—Eskalith is the brand name) to treat my bipolar disorder, we focused on its potential risks to our developing baby. If you are on another medication, your concerns will be different. Be prepared to discuss all your medications in detail with your genetic counselor. If the genetic clinic in your area does not offer preconception planning, it can refer you to one that does.

Appendix A, written by Helga Valdmanis Toriello, Ph.D., contains important information about genetic counseling. Although the information is quite technical, Dr. Toriello does a thorough job of explaining the importance of this step. She has included a table that summarizes the medications used to treat bipolar disorder and the risks to the unborn baby of anomalies (i.e., abnormalities).

Letters summarizing our genetic counseling session were sent by Dr. Toriello to Dr. Hiemenga and me. An important objective for our genetic counselor was to research lithium risks to our baby and she did her job well. She described, in detail, several abnormalities (with accompanying statistics) that could occur while taking lithium during pregnancy. Since bipolar disorder is treatable, a lesser concern to us was finding out that our children could also have the condition.

After our genetic counseling session, and especially after reading the summary letter, I felt as if the wind had been knocked out of me. Fred and I wanted to have a baby—we desperately wanted to start a family. Our odds of having a safe pregnancy and a healthy baby seemed remote. After considering all the facts, Fred and I decided that if we moved forward with our goal to have a baby, I would discontinue lithium. My next step was to learn more about that decision.

I wanted to know how long it would take before my body was lithium free. I talked with a pharmacist I knew and respected. His conclusion, based on research he obtained from Micromedex Inc. (a drug evaluation monograph), is that once lithium was discontinued, I would have a good margin of safety at twelve days.

I also discussed going off lithium in detail with my psychiatrist, Ingrid Eerdmans. (Her instructions are summarized in Chapter 4.) *It is imperative that you consult with your doctor about all medication changes.*

The NAMI Advocate (Spring/Summer 2004) reported that a 2004 study by Yonkers et al. found that:

> Because bipolar disorder emerges during young adulthood and persists throughout the lifespan, women of childbearing age are at risk for this illness. Pregnancy and delivery can influence the symptoms of bipolar disorder: pregnant women or new mothers with bipolar disorder have a sevenfold higher risk of hospital admission and a

twofold higher risk for a recurrent episode, compared with those who have not recently delivered a child or are not pregnant.

Careful planning for pregnancy can help women with bipolar disorder to optimally manage their illness to minimize their symptoms and avoid risks to the fetus. Experts suggest it is important to avoid sudden changes in medication during pregnancy, because such changes may increase side effects and risks to the fetus and also increase the risk of relapse of the illness before or after the woman gives birth. (p. 1)

I've always been one to bite off more than I can chew, and this wasn't any different. Fred and I were determined to go against the odds, conquer our fears, and bask in the joys of having a family of our own. It became not only a distant dream but a reachable destiny.

The next section was written by Jay Carter, a licensed psychologist who is certified in psychoactive substance abuse disorders by the American Psychological Association. He focuses on two important points that will help in planning your pregnancy.

Doctor's Note

BY JAY CARTER, PsyD, DABPS

Bipolar is a spectrum disorder. That means it varies in intensity depending on what genes are awry and how many genes are awry. It also varies (within spectrum limits) depending on the amount of stress that comes from the environment.

If a woman has been hospitalized in the past for bipolar disorder, I would recommend that she obtain a legal document for mental health power of attorney, which appoints someone to be her legal guardian for a specified period of time—for example, from the time she goes off medication to six weeks after she gives birth. It must be irrevocable for that period. The assignee would be her spouse, her psychiatrist, a parent, or a trusted friend. This person should be able to legally admit the assignor to a mental health unit against her (current) will, for the purpose of protecting her and her unborn child from harm and to enable a smooth transition during pregnancy.

Someone who is manic or depressed loses part of his or her executive function. The executive function is in the prefrontal lobe of the brain; it enables us to see the big picture and the context of situations. The executive function can be totally lost or lost just to the degree that one is dysfunctional in significant ways. It includes the part of the imagination that enables us to

understand the consequences of our actions. It lets us put ourselves in someone else's place and have empathy.

When the mind races six times faster than normal (as it often
does with bipolars), the cognitive (concrete) part of the brain
takes over all the brain's energy, leaving little for the executive
function in the prefrontal lobe. This can be seen in brain scans
of people who are manic. We lose our common sense, so to
speak, but usually not to the degree that it causes catastrophic,
irreversible acts to ruin our lives. One can say, "He would never
do that in his right mind" about someone who is manic.

Making the Decision

I will always remember the day that Fred and I decided we
were going to try to have a baby. It was December 7, 1990; it was
a day that continues to shape our lives.

I was a medical center representative for a pharmaceutical
company at the time. I was traveling for business, staying in a
quaint hotel overlooking Lake Michigan. I extended my stay,
Fred joined me, and we took this opportunity to focus on our
future. The apprehension and uncertainty that we had been feeling was replaced with a surge of peace and joy.

Fred comments as follows:

When Kristin and I started talking about having a baby, I was
ecstatic about being a dad. I had always thought I would like to

have children, but at the same time I was concerned for Kristin's health. We had no way of knowing how being off lithium would affect her. This was the only Kristin I knew. I felt a mixture of emotions: excitement at the idea of parenthood, but also apprehension about her well-being.

Although we were unsure of our immediate future, Fred and I were driven to begin this new chapter in our lives. Together we started breaking down this life-changing decision into manageable parts. We knew it would be safest for the baby if I didn't take lithium prior to conception and throughout the pregnancy. At the time, we believed that taking any kind of medication during that period could put our baby at risk.

I was terrified at the thought of going off lithium. Fred, too, was concerned with the risks involved for me. Would this sacrifice be too high a price to pay to have a child? I had been on lithium continuously for close to twelve years. Before I started taking it, my life had been a roller coaster. I felt as if I were trapped in a body with no control. At times I thought I was in control, but looking back, I can see that those were the times that I was manic.

My manic episodes included the following uncontrollable behavioral characteristics: a racing mind, the pressure to say everything I was thinking, an exceedingly happy mood, grandiose thoughts, and the frivolous spending of money. While hypomanic (i.e., having mild mania), I experienced some of the same symptoms, but they were not as intense.

The Bipolar Disorder Survival Guide (Miklowitz, 2002) points out that "a true hypomanic episode involves an observable change in functioning from a prior mood state. A hypomanic person sleeps less, feels mildly or moderately elated or irritable, and has racing thoughts or becomes talkative" (p. 51).

Because I refer to the term *hypomanic* throughout the book, I'm giving an example of how it affects me. There are times even today when I know that I'm hypomanic. It's often triggered by a self-imposed goal. My hypomanic symptoms include intense stress, agitation, and anxiety. The compulsion I feel to complete my task is all consuming. Although I give myself deadlines to stop working, I rarely stop on my own. The pressure is there to continue. Time passes quickly, and I keep on working. Once I stop, my thoughts are still racing. My mind and body feel like a revved-up car engine with no hope of running out of gas.

During my depressed periods I felt lonely, isolated, and hopeless. I didn't want to open the door to mania or depression as a result of our decision for me to discontinue lithium. However, I did realize it would be temporary.

Our primary goal was to increase our chance of having a healthy baby. We knew that this would involve making some lifestyle changes. Our initial challenge was to identify the areas in my life that were stressful. The first thing that came to mind was my career.

Fred and I knew that I would have to quit my job. My career was extremely technical and stressful. I knew I wouldn't be able to effectively fulfill the responsibilities of a pharmaceutical representative once I discontinued lithium. Also, I had an extensive territory that required overnight travel and long hours on the road. I didn't know if I would be able to drive safely or communicate effectively with others. Thus I could not perform my job competently once I went off lithium. The stress level would surely send me into a manic episode.

So Fred and I developed a plan.

The Importance of Journaling

It was crucial that I record each stage of my pregnancy. Writing in my "pregnancy journal" was one of the most effective ways to monitor myself from preconception through postpartum. I started writing in my pregnancy journal when Fred and I made the decision to have a baby. I knew it was important to record how we felt about this decision before I discontinued lithium. Writing in my pregnancy journal served many purposes.

Once I quit taking lithium, my journal helped me to maintain control; this is the antithesis of being off lithium. I didn't think I'd have much control over my racing mind and moods once I stopped taking the drug. My thoughts and feelings made more sense when I recorded them. It was a way to compartmentalize the utter chaos buzzing around in my mind.

Once I wrote them down, I had a sense of temporary peace. This was my way of "reeling myself in" when necessary. Writing my feelings down also helped me to manage and cope with stress and agitation. My journal was always there, and it immediately became part of my support system. It was my "safe place"—my sounding board.

Recording specific dates helped me to put my life in perspective. If I had not documented dates, everyday events and milestones would have become one gigantic blur. It was another way in which I sought to exert control when I felt it slipping away. For many bipolars, dates are a touchstone in our mind-set.

I recorded and monitored the schedule that Dr. Ingrid Eerdmans, my psychiatrist, recommended for discontinuing lithium. The act of writing helped me to control hypomanic behaviors. When I was depressed and worried excessively, writing helped me to express and understand those feelings. Keeping track of my thoughts and progress helped me to see myself throughout this challenging time. My pregnancy journal kept me on track and validated me.

Journaling was not new for me. I had kept a daily diary from ages ten to twenty. Even during college, I occasionally wrote in a journal to help sort out my emotions. Writing has always been a safe haven for my feelings and thoughts that others might not have understood.

I realize, however, that not everyone wants or is able to keep a written journal. That's okay; there are several ways to journal. Using a computer or an audiotape to help manage your bipolar symptoms can also help you to organize your thoughts and record your progress. Ongoing communication with your support team (i.e., partner, medical professionals, friends, and family) is another effective tool.

In this book, I focus on keeping a written journal because it worked so well for me—especially in managing my first pregnancy. During my second pregnancy, I used my calendar to supplement my journal. Use a method of journaling that works for you.

For my first pregnancy, I started writing down my feelings in December, as soon as we had made the decision. It was as if I were trying to validate myself. At that point I didn't realize that my journal would serve as a lifeline prior to conception, during pregnancy, and after the birth of our baby. As you can imagine, bipolar journals can be very wordy. All those details I felt compelled to write about went on and on. Throughout this book you will find italicized excerpts from my journal. Many journal entries have been omitted—for your benefit (unless you're like my dad and enjoy an occasional nap while reading).

December 16: Fred and I are thrilled about trying to have a baby. There's no question in my mind that this is the right thing to do. Also, the timing is right!

On December 19, 1990, I handed my division manager my resignation letter, effective January 2, 1991. To say that I was reluctant to tell him is, at best, an understatement. I was so scared that I was trembling. When he read the letter, the look on his face broke my heart. I felt as if I had blindsided him, that I was letting him down.

The worst part was that I could not give him the real reason for my decision. I told him I was leaving for "personal reasons." It was difficult to look him in the eye and not level with him.

I am a straightforward person and felt guilty and deceitful for not being truthful, but I believed that it was necessary to remain a "closet" bipolar. Our meeting ended amicably, and I was relieved to have that hurdle behind me.

December 19: I am proud of my accomplishments as a pharmaceutical representative. I feel excellent about my decision to leave. The pressure of this job is enormous. I feel as if a weight has been lifted from my shoulders. I am now free to concentrate on our next step.

I realize that this journal entry contradicts how I was feeling during the meeting with my manager. I referred to this entry whenever I felt twinges of remorse about leaving my career.

Fred and I knew that it was important for me to work part time. After I graduated from college, a significant part of my identity and self-worth was bound up in my career. A job also gave me a feeling of achievement. Financially, it was not necessary for me to work, but contributing to the household income had always been important to me; it gave me a feeling of autonomy. I was afraid that now I'd have trouble cutting back on my spending, and I knew that discontinuing lithium would make me more prone to shopping sprees.

Working part time was therefore a logical decision for our situation. You need to assess what is best for you and your family.

Stress is a precursor to bipolar symptoms. For example, stress causes my mind to race. When my mind is racing, it does not stop; I am thinking continuously. During conversations with others, it's extremely difficult for me to concentrate on what they're saying. My mind is often occupied with several sidebar conversations. Sometimes I try to think of ways to speed up the conversation because it's painful to converse at what I perceive as a slow pace in others. It is also difficult to act as if none of this is going on. Others are usually unaware of the turmoil that is going on in my head. Over the years, self-discipline has enabled me to appear normal when my mind is racing. While I was off the medication and I became exceedingly revved up due to stress, I could no longer conceal my racing mind. (I will explain this more throughout the book.)

Trying to sleep at night can be frustrating. Despite the fact I am tired, my mind is not; it's wound up tight. I feel as if my mind is not connected to me. It keeps thinking and thinking, and I have no control over it. Bipolar symptoms make it hard to sleep, and lack of sleep increases bipolar symptoms. It's a vicious cycle.

Fred and I believed that my working part time would meet our objectives while decreasing my stress level, so I answered an ad in the newspaper for a part-time marketing consultant for a trade show. I interviewed for the job and was hired. My primary responsibilities included contacting business owners and managers and selling the benefits of participating in an area trade show.

December 19 [continued]: *I'm looking forward to starting my new job as a marketing consultant in January. Everything's falling into place. The conditions involving this decision couldn't be better. I have support from Fred, my family, and friends!*

Three weeks later I wrote a journal entry that demonstrated the intense emotions and challenges I experienced as a result of giving up my career as a medical center representative. Writing down my feelings helped me to actively work through my apprehension and anxiety. Although my job had been demanding and stressful, it was also gratifying. Now I felt as if I were fading into a shadow of the competent person I once was. It really scared me.

January 6, 1991: On December 28, I drove my company car and all the company belongings to my former division manager's house [he lived about fifty-five miles from me, so I had plenty of time to grieve the loss of my career]. *I've been sad and depressed about resigning since December 19. I was devastated during the ride back from Lansing that day. I felt empty and cried throughout the ride home. The reasons I'm feeling this way are as follows: (1) A large portion of my self-esteem is derived from my prior job. (2) I liked being a medical center representative—I really liked my job! (3) Calling my key contacts to tell them that I was leaving (especially at my open-heart hospitals) was extremely difficult. I wanted to share my exciting news with them but knew it wouldn't be appropriate. When asked, I believed I had to tell them I was leaving for personal reasons. The majority of them told me they'd miss me and that I was/am a very good representative: dependable, knowledgeable, and professional. I was flattered by their comments. I feel a connection to some of them; I feel as if they're my accounts. I provided them with excellent service—took good care of them. (4) I feel as if I'm permanently closing the door to a career that's become a huge part of my identity and my life. (5) I'm going to have to adjust to not making as much money. I'm not worried about that now, but it will be something that I'll have to work on in the future.*

On the positive side it sure feels great to have my "life" back again. I'm looking forward to spending more quality time with Fred, cooking [it's funny that I mentioned cooking, because my family and friends know that I make quick and simple meals], *working out, and spending time with friends. No more overnights, driving 600–900 miles per week, or extensive planning and paperwork. I started my new job January 3. I look at this job as temporary. I know it won't utilize my skills or challenge me like my previous job. However, this position is perfect for me now. It will be interesting to see if I'll be able to work once I go off lithium.*

A week later I acknowledge the frustrations of my new job and give myself a pep talk.

January 14: There is a lot of potential (considering it's part time and flexible) to make money in this position. Try not to get discouraged—I know that I'll be closing lots of sales soon. Keep working at it each day; I'm certain my efforts will pay off. This position is temporary for me. It's a vehicle to keep me employed during this time, to enable me to make some money, have a positive focus, and keep up my self-esteem (professionally). All of these things will help Fred and me to reach our goals.

Fred and I didn't spend much time discussing the question "What if we have a child who is later diagnosed as bipolar?" If we had had a crystal ball that told us that both of our children would have bipolar disorder, we still would have moved forward with our decision. It wasn't a concern for us. Fred and I were confident that we could overcome that challenge if it happened—and it did. Katherine Kay was diagnosed with bipolar disorder in 2004—

but that's another story, literally. I have truly been embracing my bipolar condition since my college days. For me it has been a blessing in disguise.

We Decide to Have a Second Baby

Our decision to try to conceive a second baby was easier than the first decision. Fred and I kept an open mind for two years while I was back on lithium. After the birth of our first baby on December 8, 1991, and before resuming lithium, I was obsessing about having only one child. (Chapter 9 elaborates on my thought process at that volatile time. Decisions of this magnitude should not be made while you're off medication.)

Before you resume medication, concentrate on your new baby. There's no reason to think about having another at this point. Fred and I knew when the time was right. We waited until we had the same burning desire we did the first time. We had a better idea of what to expect and were confident that we could manage each phase of the pregnancy. It never occurred to us that I might not be able to conceive a second time, but if that had been the case, we would have accepted it with disappointment.

A friend and former coworker mentioned to me that her company was interested in hiring an experienced pharmaceutical representative. This occurred while we were thinking of baby number two.

November 23, 1993 [I had not written in my journal since I resumed taking lithium nine weeks after Katherine was born]:

Fred and I decided to have another baby. Katherine would surely enjoy a brother or sister.

December 2: I'll let my friend know that I'm not interested in a full-time pharmaceutical position with another company. Fred and I seriously considered the pros and cons of having a second baby, and our priorities were crystal clear.

As part of the decision-making process, we agreed it would be best if I had a career with flexible hours. I decided to study to become an investment advisor representative. My father is in the financial and estate planning business. He was thrilled with my decision. I was confident that I could start the licensing and training process during my pregnancy.

This was a pivotal decision, because I needed something significant to concentrate on (above and beyond my husband and wonderful daughter) during my pregnancy. It was also important for me to work at a career that expanded my mind, offered challenges, and enabled me to help others.

Everyone has a unique set of circumstances that must be considered. It's crucial to have the support of your partner, because he or she has to help you through this potentially difficult time. Discuss some specific ways to help decrease your stress level (e.g., sharing in the household responsibilities). Extra patience is also important.

Fred says the following:

Once Kristin and I decided to have a baby, I knew that I had to help her as much as possible during this unpredictable time. Being off her medication would be a huge challenge for both of us. I felt that any way I could reduce stress in her life and reinforce positive activities, such as walking, playing cards, or enjoying a movie together, would help keep her on track.

Consider the challenges you might encounter in your relationships when experiencing possible mania and/or depression. Refer to Chapters 3 and 4 for specific suggestions to help monitor your behavior changes. It is imperative that all major decisions be made *prior* to discontinuing medication or once medication is *resumed.* This is important because significant decisions require judgment and detailed planning, both of which can be impaired while you are off medication.

It might benefit you and your partner to have a written plan that describes how you are going to make the necessary lifestyle changes to accomplish your goal of having a healthy baby.

Let's take another look at the decision to work outside the home. The financial consequences of decreasing your hours, changing jobs to work part time, or quitting your job can impact your ability to pay your bills. That's an important consideration. If you decide to try to work at your current job, and if you choose to go off medication, there is a chance that your stress level will increase dramatically, possibly causing you to get fired or quit in a manic moment. Write down a contingency plan so that you are prepared if this occurs. For example, if your income is necessary to pay the bills and you do quit your job, you might decide to stop trying to conceive, resume taking your medication, and look for another job.

Talk with your psychiatrist and health care provider about the best plan of action concerning possible medication changes. I had an ob-gyn; you might choose to use a nurse-midwife, family practitioner, nurse practitioner, or physician's assistant. Do not deviate from these professionals' recommendations; they are the experts. Ongoing communication with them is important.

If you are going to discontinue your medication prior to conception, decide on a specific length of time to try this. If you adjust well during this time, you might feel comfortable staying off your meds. However, it can take years for some women to get pregnant, if at all. As part of your written plan, be sure to follow the advice of your partner, psychiatrist, and ob-gyn to resume medication if your bipolar symptoms warrant it. You should also discuss with your physician(s) the option of resuming medication during your pregnancy if your life is at risk because of your bipolar symptoms.

Writing down a time limit to be off medication (while you are feeling stable) can help to decrease any disappointment or guilt you experience if you have trouble conceiving. During a manic or depressive episode, it's difficult to make good decisions. Your ob-gyn will be able to provide you with suggestions for how to decrease the time from conception to restarting medication.

SUMMARY

Women who are affected with bipolar disorder (and their partners) have several things to consider while deciding if they should
attempt to conceive. It is also important to do the following:

- Educate yourself and your partner on bipolar disorder
  (see Chapter 10).

- Consult with your psychiatrist and ob-gyn.

- Schedule an appointment with a genetic counselor for
  preconception planning.

- Research the risks to your baby and yourself.

- Formulate a written plan to guide you through the
  pregnancy process.

- Prepare for lifestyle and/or career changes to decrease
  stress levels.

- Implement the changes.

- Keep a journal to document your progress and thought
  process.

The next step is to plan for pregnancy.

Chapter 2

Planning for a Healthy Pregnancy

The period in which we planned for my pregnancy was a time of excitement and anticipation. Fred and I hoped that I would get pregnant as quickly as possible so that the length of time from discontinuing lithium to conceiving would be minimal. I didn't want to be off lithium any longer than necessary.

Your ob-gyn is an excellent resource for conception and pregnancy issues. Dr. Hiemenga, my ob-gyn, gave me a basal temperature chart to use to determine when I was ovulating. This chart was an effective tool for increasing my chances of conception because it kept me aware of my body's monthly cyclical changes. In December 1990, I started filling it in each day, and it gave me a feeling of control. A pattern developed: I noticed that ovulation occurred around the time that I felt monthly cramping. It was usually low on one side of my abdomen.

Dr. Hiemenga also provided us with additional tips to increase my chances of becoming pregnant. These are included in Appendix B.

An Internet article, "Planning a Pregnancy: Getting Ready for Baby" (www.realsavvymoms.com), provides the following helpful information to complement what your ob-gyn will review with you:

> If you are planning to become pregnant, taking certain steps can help reduce risks to both you and your baby. Proper health before deciding to become pregnant is almost as important as maintaining a healthy body during pregnancy. This is because the first 12 weeks of pregnancy is a very sensitive time. The risk of miscarriage is the greatest. In addition, all of the baby's organs are developing, so the risk of birth defects is also the greatest. By the time most women realize that they are pregnant, this important time has already passed. By planning ahead, you can affect important factors in your lifestyle that can help prevent potential problems. Steps that you should take the ensure you have a healthy pregnancy and baby should include a pre-pregnancy exam, a smoking cessation program, a proper diet with vitamins, an exercise and weight management program, medical management of pre-existing conditions, a conscious effort to prevent birth defects, infection control, and staying away from harmful substances.

Physical exercise is also beneficial while you are pregnant. The March of Dimes advises the following in its website article "Fitness for Two" (www.marchofdimes.com):

For many women, exercise is an important part of their lives, and they want to continue their exercise programs during pregnancy. In most cases, they can. Numerous studies have demonstrated that, in low-risk pregnancies, moderate or even vigorous exercise is safe for the baby. The American College of Obstetricians and Gynecologists (ACOG) now recommends that most pregnant women participate in 30 minutes or more of moderate exercise on most, if not all, days of the week.

Regular exercise leads to improved fitness for pregnant women, just as it does for all women and men. It helps keep the heart, mind and entire body healthy. Exercise helps prevent health problems like heart disease, high blood pressure, diabetes, osteoporosis (bone loss), anxiety, depression and, possibly, some forms of cancer. For the pregnant woman, it can ease many common discomforts of pregnancy, such as constipation, backache, fatigue and varicose veins. Regular exercise also may help prevent pregnancy-related forms of diabetes and high blood pressure. Fit women may be able to cope better with labor and have a faster recovery after delivery.

Pregnant women who have not exercised regularly should consider gradually increasing their activities or starting a mild exercise program to reap some of these health benefits. However, all pregnant women should check with a health care provider before starting or continuing exercise. Most women will be able to maintain their exercise program throughout pregnancy, although some may need to modify their activities. Women who don't exercise regularly can obtain many of its health benefits by following an active lifestyle. Past recommendations stated that a person needed to exercise continuously for about 30 minutes at least three times a week to obtain health benefits. However, current recommendations from the Centers for Disease Control and Prevention (CDC) say that short bouts of activity (at least 10 minutes each) several times a day also are effective. . . .

Exercise has additional benefits for women with bipolar disorder. Throughout pregnancy, exercise provided me with a release that helped me to manage my bipolar symptoms. I have exercised regularly since I was a young teen for two primary reasons: It makes me feel good, and it helps me maintain my weight (I love to eat!). The health benefits are a bonus.

Exercise helps me to maintain a positive mental attitude. Even during times of depression, regular exercise gave me a sense of accomplishment and often made me feel better. During hypomanic periods, it helped to quiet my racing mind. Exercise is an effective way to channel or burn excess energy.

While Fred and I were in the planning stages of pregnancy, I continued my exercise routine, which consisted of weight lifting, aerobics, walking, and toning exercises. My goal was to get some form of exercise four to six times per week. It's important to make it a habit.

To keep track of my progress, I kept a monthly chart of all the exercise I completed each day. This gave me a snapshot of my exercise routine. Prior to conception, during pregnancy, and postpartum I referred to these summaries to help monitor the amount of exercise I was getting.

Moderation is the key. It's difficult to exhibit moderation of any kind when you're hypomanic or manic. Knowing that I have a tendency to exaggerate any type of behavior or habit, I felt good that I could quickly summarize my exercise. It was especially comforting because I would be discontinuing lithium soon. I knew that I would give up some control when I went off my medication (and, for example, exercise too much). Keeping this chart was my way of regaining that control. I also realized that my husband would let me know if I was overdoing it, and I wouldn't be able to say to him, "I'm not exercising too much," because my records would indicate otherwise. Fred made the following comments about exercise:

> Kristin and I have both been very health conscious since we have known each other. We actually met after running a 25K race! I knew that she would continue to exercise during her pregnancy to stay healthy. I felt like I had a new role in her life, like a trainer or coach—to encourage her to continue to exercise, but not let her overdo it.

I knew that it might be helpful to refer to my exercise chart while talking with my ob-gyn. The chart also provided a way for me to monitor my exercise as I decreased the intensity of my workouts in the late months of pregnancy.

The March of Dimes article "During Your Pregnancy: Stress" (www.marchofdimes.com) highlights additional ways to avoid or decrease stress in your life:

What you need to know: Pregnancy is a stressful time for many women. You may be feeling happy, sad and scared—all at the same time. It's okay to feel like you do. Very high levels of stress may contribute to preterm birth or low birth weight in full-term babies, however, so you should try to learn how to cope with it.

What you can do: Recognize that you do indeed feel stressed. Accepting the fact you are stressed and identifying the situations that cause you stress are the first steps in helping reduce it. You can also help reduce your stress by:

- Eating regularly and nutritiously and drinking lots of water.
- Resting when you can—and when your body needs it.
- Exercising (with your health care provider's okay).
- Relaxing by meditating, listening to music or writing in a journal.
- Resisting any urges to drink alcohol, smoke or take herbal products or drugs (except those prescribed by your health care provider).
- Staying away from stressful people and stressful situations, when possible.
- Talking—to your partner, friends, relatives, health care professionals, and your employer. If you feel overwhelmed, talk with a trained counselor or other mental health professional.
- Going to all your prenatal care appointments. This will give you the reassurance that everything is okay with your baby or let your health care provider know about a problem while there is still time to do something about it. You'll feel less stressed because you know you are doing the best for your baby.

Prior to making any changes in your medication, it's important to address unresolved emotional problems, baggage, or concerns—anything that can come back to haunt you. I'm writing from experience. During my second pregnancy, I struggled with an unresolved, troublesome issue that I thought had been buried. I had no idea that it would repeat itself like a movie rerun, over and over again in my racing mind, as I tried to sleep at night. I couldn't get away from it. Now, during the planning stage, is the time to address unresolved emotional problems and worries. Talk with someone from your support network.

There is another important issue you need to explore when planning a pregnancy: Are you going to breastfeed your baby? Discuss the risks and benefits of your decision with your doctors and your partner. Restarting medication after delivery might be the best decision for you, and you often can't breastfeed if you're taking medication because the drug will pass through your milk to the baby. Even if you decide ahead of time to breastfeed, it's okay to change your mind once the baby is born. Resuming your medication might become necessary and be in the best interest of you and your baby. Keep in mind that the chances of postpartum depression are higher for bipolar women.

If you do decide to breastfeed, before you go off your medication you should write a plan of action that includes the following:

1. Understanding why you want to breastfeed your baby and how important it is to you.

2. Talking to your doctors about medications that can be used safely while nursing.

3. Contacting local hospitals while you're pregnant to get information about (a) prenatal breastfeeding classes, (b) breastfeeding support groups to attend after your baby is born, and (c) a certified lactation consultant who can advise you if you have to abruptly discontinue breastfeeding and need to wean your baby quickly.

4. Knowing when you should listen to your doctors, partner, family, and trusted friends for guidance because you are unable to realize that you need to resume your medication.

5. Dealing with any feelings of guilt for discontinuing breastfeeding. Know that you are doing the right thing, and focus on the future—your health and your ability to care for your baby. You cannot take care of anyone else if you haven't taken care of yourself.

SUMMARY

Planning for a healthy pregnancy is especially important for those who have bipolar disorder. The following steps will help you to succeed:

- Discuss with your ob-gyn how to decrease the time it takes to conceive, so you can minimize the duration of changes in your medication.

- Prior to decreasing, changing, or discontinuing your medication, address unresolved emotional problems or issues and explore the possibility of breastfeeding.

- Implement your ob-gyn's recommendations.

- Keep a pregnancy journal (as described in Chapter 1) to monitor yourself from preconception to postpartum. This journal will help you to process and track your thoughts and feelings and to control racing thoughts.

- After consulting with your ob-gyn, start or continue an exercise program to help manage bipolar symptoms and reduce stress. Keep an exercise chart.

Chapter 3

Preparing to
Go Off Medication

I was diagnosed with bipolar disorder in April 1979 and immediately began taking lithium. I didn't stop taking it even when I felt better (i.e., became stabilized), because I understood that bipolar disorder is a chemical imbalance for which I would need medication for the rest of my life. As I prepared to discontinue lithium to become pregnant, I was terrified. Can you imagine going off a medication that has sustained your sanity? I hadn't experienced the intense, ongoing symptoms of mania and depression in more than ten years. I had to prepare myself to open up old wounds.

One of my greatest concerns about discontinuing lithium was that perhaps my mind would turn to mush. I knew that when I was either manic or depressed (which was inevitable), I would get so caught up in the moment that I might forget I am a worthwhile, intelligent person.

Looking ahead, I decided that it was necessary to hold on to my intelligence and confidence as long as possible. I wrote out a short presentation that I shared with physicians and nurses while I was employed by the pharmaceutical company. I summarized the benefits of using Inocor (amrinone) to treat congestive heart failure and to help wean patients off the bypass machine after open-heart surgery. I wrote this presentation in my journal on January 14, 1991, as I was mentally preparing to discontinue lithium. (It might sound technical and boring to you, but writing it helped me to hold on to my self-worth.) This entry reminded me that once I resumed medication, I could and would again be able to tackle difficult tasks with ease.

January 14, 1991: Inocor is a positive inotrope with vasodilitory properties. Inocor increases cardiac index and reduces pulmonary capillary wedge pressure (PCWP) without increasing heart rate or the potential for arrhythmias.

MVO_2 [myocardial oxygen consumption] *generally stays the same or decreases because systolic wall tension is decreased. That's especially beneficial for ischemic patients, or patients with coronary artery disease.*

In those situations where you have a patient on Dobutamine for forty-eight to seventy-two hours, tachyphalaxis, or drug tolerance, often occurs. Some physicians have told me that in some cases they titrate the dose up to 10–20 mcg/kg/min [micrograms per kilograms per minute] *to maintain the initial efficacy—heart rate tends to go up, and the potential for arrhythmias increases. There is no documented evidence of tachyphalaxis with Inocor. Efficacy is maintained throughout treatment.*

The difference in mechanism of action between Inocor and Dobutamine is important. Inocor is a phosphodiesterase III inhibitor. Patients experience tachyphalaxis with Dobutamine because of beta downregulation.

It's also important to remember that when you administer Dobutamine to a patient who has been on beta blockers, you may not get the total response because the beta receptor sites are blocked. This is not a problem with Inocor (because it works through a different mechanism of action).

My career as a pharmaceutical representative required technical expertise and the ability to communicate the benefits of the products I represented. Knowing that I possessed this ability gave me the confidence that once my medication was resumed, these attributes would return.

Summarizing this presentation was therapeutic for me. I couldn't write the words down quickly enough. This increased my self-confidence. I knew that once lithium was discontinued, I could refer to my journal and read this entry. It would remind me of what I am capable of being and doing.

Use this idea; adapt it to your situation. You might want to summarize your achievements. Write down anything that makes you feel good about yourself. Take it a step further and gather some special items that mean a lot to you.

For example, fill a shoe box with positive reminders of your life prior to discontinuing, reducing the dosage of, or changing your medication. Have some fun with this. Refer to the shoe box any time you need to feel validated. Here are some ideas:

- Photographs of happy times
- Cards or letters from people who mean a lot to you
- Awards or other recognition for something you've accomplished
- Reminders of goals that you set for yourself and achieved
- A letter written to yourself during the times you felt best

By filling the box with reminders of your happy and good life, you will have physical evidence of how your life was prior to medication changes, and in difficult times it will give you the hope of knowing that you will be like that again.

Fred made the following comments:

I made up my mind I that I would help any way I could. I was hoping we could get through the first trimester so that afterwards she could possibly go on a low dose of lithium.

I wasn't sure how I would handle Kristin being off lithium. She gave me some examples of her behavior before she began taking it, and of course I didn't want to see her thrown back into that turmoil. I was apprehensive and concerned about seeing this side of Kristin take full force. Kristin's health was my priority. However, she was convinced she could handle it and thought that once she became pregnant, the pregnancy hormones might actually help her cope.

Mental Health America (www.mentalhealthamerica.net) describes bipolar signs and symptoms this way:

Bipolar disorder is often difficult to recognize and diagnose. It causes a person to have a high level of energy, grandiose thoughts or ideas, and impulsive or reckless behavior. These symptoms may feel good to a person, which may lead to denial that there is a problem. Another reason bipolar disorder is difficult to diagnose is that its symptoms may appear to be part of another illness or attributed to other problems, such as substance abuse, poor school performance, or trouble in the workplace.

Symptoms of Mania

The symptoms of mania, which can last up to three months if untreated, include:

- Excessive energy, activity, restlessness, racing thoughts, and rapid talking
- Denial that anything is wrong
- Extreme "high" or euphoric feelings—a person may feel "on top of the world" and nothing, including bad news or tragic events, can change this "happiness."
- Easily irritated or distracted
- Decreased need for sleep—an individual may last for days with little or no sleep without feeling tired.
- Unrealistic beliefs in one's ability and powers—a person may experience feelings of exaggerated confidence or unwarranted optimism. This can lead to overly ambitious work plans and the belief that nothing can stop him or her from accomplishing any task.

- Uncharacteristically poor judgment—a person may make poor decisions which may lead to unrealistic involvement in activities, meetings and deadlines, reckless driving, spending sprees, and foolish business ventures.

- Sustained period of behavior that is different from usual—a person may dress and/or act differently than he or she usually does, become a collector of various items, become indifferent to personal grooming, become obsessed with writing, or experience delusions.

- Unusual sexual drive

- Abuse of drugs, particularly cocaine, alcohol or sleeping medications

- Provocative, intrusive or aggressive behavior—a person may become enraged or paranoid if his or her grand ideas are stopped or excessive social plans are refused."

Dr. Eerdmans defines a manic episode as an elevated mood occurring with three or more of the above symptoms each day, for one week or longer. If the mood is irritable, as opposed to elevated, four additional symptoms must be present.

Mental Health America further notes:

Symptoms of Depression

Some people experience periods of normal mood and behavior following a manic phase; however, the depressive phase will eventually appear. Symptoms of depression include:

- Persistent sad, anxious or empty mood
- Sleeping too much or too little, middle-of-the-night or early morning waking
- Reduced appetite and weight loss or increased appetite and weight gain
- Loss of interest or pleasure in activities, including sex
- Irritability or restlessness
- Difficulty concentrating, remembering or making decisions
- Fatigue or loss of energy
- Persistent physical symptoms that don't respond to treatment (such as chronic pain or digestive disorders)
- Thoughts of death or suicide, including suicide attempts
- Feeling guilty, hopeless, worthless

Dr. Eerdmans defines a depressive episode as having five or more of the above symptoms lasting most of the day, nearly every day, for a period of two weeks or longer.

The psychiatrist who diagnosed me with bipolar disorder (referred to then as manic-depressive illness) had given me a pamphlet describing manic and depressive symptoms. I had not looked at it or read about bipolar disorder since that time (1979). Prior to discontinuing lithium, I needed to establish a way to monitor my behavior so that I could manage it.

On January 5, 1991, I made a list in my journal of my previous bipolar symptoms. Explanations follow most of them. You'll notice that many feed off each other and are connected.

My Symptoms of Mania

Racing mind. Multiple thoughts came at me like a persistent, hard rain and sometimes felt as explosive as lightning bolts. My racing mind rarely slowed down. It was like a separate entity that was impossible to tame. These thoughts occurred both while I was by myself and during conversations with others. Being alone with my thoughts was overwhelming and exhausting. For example, I frequently wrote in my diary (or notebook, if I had more to say than the limited space my diary provided) to help me organize and "make sense" of my thoughts and feelings. I felt that they were racing at the speed of light; writing them down was my lifeline and escape prior to my diagnosis.

Compulsion to talk. My compulsion to talk was a result of my racing mind. My mental gatekeeper—the discernment that I used to decide what to say and what to keep to myself—had malfunctioned. One of my favorite activities as a young teen was to hang out with an older, "cool" cousin. I loved to ride to her apartment with her after church. The two of us would have lunch together and visit by the swimming pool. It was "girl talk" at its best—or so I thought. Years later she told me that there were times that I talked nonstop. It was therapeutic for me, yet anything but relaxing for her. I had no idea that words were coming out of my mouth like items coming off a production line.

Poor listening due to racing mind; difficulty concentrating and focusing. Can you imagine trying to understand others when your mind is competing for the same attention that you're desperately trying to give them? It felt like a constant tug-of-war. Focusing during classes at school was impossible. It was as if the bridge required to convey the teachers' messages to my brain were permanently blocked. The information would not penetrate. I didn't realize the extent to which this was happening because it had become so much a part of my everyday world.

Driving too fast. I was a fast and erratic driver. I used to ask my younger brother if I drove as well as my dad and older brother. Diplomatically, he would reply, "If a professional race-car driver is a ten, Dad and Michael are probably an eight. You are a five or six." He was generous.

Conceitedness. I graduated from modeling school in October 1977. For two years I had a modeling job with a well-known clothing store. When it was my turn to walk down the runway, I believed that I had an intense connection with the audience. I effortlessly made a connection with each person (or so I thought) by looking directly into his or her eyes. I felt confident and beautiful. The positive feedback I received fueled my confidence and turned it into conceitedness.

Self-absorbed, in my own world, "Kristin-oriented." At times I felt as if the world should revolve around me. If it didn't, I would consciously manipulate the situation and my surroundings to suit me. When I was a teenager, my family went on several ski vacations to New Hampshire. The last time we went, I had no interest in skiing with my family or the family we were visiting, so I would frequently venture off by myself. I was more interested in spending time in the lodge than in skiing. My goal was to meet cute boys! I might have just described a typical teenage scenario, but in my case it was exaggerated. I even told my parents that I hurt my ankle so I could "rest it" in the lodge. I left no room for compromise and wasn't aware of how I was perceived by others.

Speaking my mind with no regard for how my message was perceived. As I reflected back, trying to think of a specific example, I immediately assumed that I didn't say things to hurt others. I must have been in denial, for then a vivid memory surfaced of which I'm ashamed. I was riding up the chairlift with my mom during the previously mentioned ski trip. I don't remember what I said to her, but I'll never forget her response to my cutting words. She burst into tears. I felt so ashamed (and, at the same time, unaware that I had said anything hurtful). I was disrespectful and cruel. Had she not started crying, I would not have had the ability to understand how she perceived what I said to her.

Impulsive and excessive shopping. Prior to age fourteen I was trustworthy and conscientious in all aspects of my life. Actually, I was a Goody Two-Shoes. Knowing that, my parents lent me a couple of credit cards for clothes, feeling confident that I would be responsible and pay them back. During November and December of 1978, however, I spent $600. I recorded the exact dates and dollar amounts in my diary for each shopping spree, then wrote "Charge it!" I recall walking into a store and selecting whatever I wanted. Nothing was too good for me. I was as addicted to buying clothes as a smoker is addicted to nicotine.

Once my mom realized that I had a new wardrobe, she went with me to return everything that had not been worn. Of course, I had to return the credit cards as well. I was upset, but I obediently returned both because intellectually I knew that my purchases were exorbitant.

My mother had the following recollection of this event:

> When Kristin's dad and I lent her the credit cards, we assumed that good judgment would prevail, as it had in the past. Because we were busy parents of three children and had lives of our own, the month flew by before I realized that Kristin was wearing too many new outfits. Imagine my shock when I looked in her closet and found more outfits hanging, with the tags still attached. Tough love initiated the trip back to several stores, where I watched as Kristin returned the clothes.

Lack of judgment, risk-taking behavior, lying to avoid getting into trouble, promiscuity, other inappropriate behavior, and lack of awareness of my actions, total cluelessness. These characteristics often occurred simultaneously, with lack of judgment being the catalyst. The following example occurred during the peak of my mania while I was in New Hampshire. One evening, I made a collect phone call to a friend back home. I initiated an engaging, flirtatious conversation with a young male phone operator. I asked him if he knew of any parties in the area. He said he'd meet me at the corner of a nearby street that evening, and we'd go to a party together. I didn't have a clue about how dangerous this could be. Prior to leaving, my parents found out about my tightly woven "plan" (lie). My dad was furious! I had never seen him so mad. Seeing his response helped me to realize that I was out of control.

Despite this lack of understanding, I thought I knew exactly what I was doing. In general, when my parents confronted me about some of the intricate lies I told them, I vehemently denied any wrongdoing (even as I looked directly into their eyes). Lying to avoid discipline felt as natural as breathing. What a contrast from the honesty and integrity I had cultivated prior to the onset of bipolar disorder and again when I began taking lithium.

Limited common sense. I thought nothing of riding in a car with friends during a blizzard to go to a concert. I had looked forward to going for weeks, and nothing was going to stop me. It never occurred to me that I might end up in a ditch wearing a fashionable coat (but no hat or gloves) and high heels. My arrogance and lack of judgment took control of my life. My dad called my friend's house just as we were about to leave and demanded that I come home immediately. I was tempted to disobey him, but he was so adamant that I grudgingly acceded to his judgment and went home.

Limited street sense. Prior to learning how to drive, I was oblivious to my surroundings while riding in a car. East, west, north, and south were not part of my realm of understanding. I realize this can be common for teenagers who are not affected with bipolar disorder, but according to my older brother, I thought that I was invincible and could manipulate my way out of any type of trouble.

Enormous amounts of energy. My leg would constantly move back and forth, and I enjoyed playing the card game "Nutsey" (triple solitaire that is played against an opponent)—I found it very calming! For most people, playing Nutsey would not have a soothing effect. I liked it because it was fast and required my attention to be diverted to several areas simultaneously. No one ever consistently beat me. I first realized how good at it I was when I was a child and played it with my aunt and uncle, who used to have Nutsey tournaments with their friends. I went through my cards like a dealer in Vegas.

Difficulty sleeping. My continuous stream of rapid thoughts kept me awake. I didn't even feel tired. My nighttime activities included the following:

- A strong desire to stay up until 3:00 or 4:00 A.M. to write—it helped to ease my racing mind and release the pressure I felt. It was also an outlet for my heightened creativity. I wrote in my diary or my notebook or wrote letters. In March 1979 (one month before my diagnosis), I wrote the following: "Commandments for you, Kristin . . . abide by them and continue to separate your dreams from your REALITIES!!" This list of rules to live by was similar to the Ten Commandments, but I personalized them. I still have these self-imposed rules, and they're proof of my attempt to recapture my life.

- Writing letters to relatives and friends that were inappropriate—many of them I decided not to send (thankfully).

The same night I wrote the "Commandments for Kristin," I wrote a bizarre letter to both sets of grandparents. My letters were overly affectionate, but it was evident that my thoughts were coming from my heart. In one letter I told my grandma and grandpa to expect a letter from me at least once a month. They were to check their mailbox on the second day of every month. I told my other grandparents that they would receive a letter on the twenty-seventh day of every month. I have no idea where those dates came from, but I was very precise. Every inch of the stationery and both envelopes were covered with writing or "art." My heart was in the right place, but my mind was not. I did not mail either letter, and I still have them.

Messy, almost illegible, writing. Some of my diary and notebook entries are difficult to decipher; this was unusual because I had always taken pride in my penmanship. The more manic I felt, the larger and sloppier my writing became. Writing with codes and symbols was common. Parts of my diaries are covered with racing, haphazard thoughts. The turbulence I experienced jumps off each page.

Keeping my private papers stashed under my bed. My room was always neat. However, one look under my bed indicated the horrible turmoil in my life. Years after I began taking lithium, my mom told me that she knew about the unorganized papers and unsent letters piled there. As I look back, I see that I might have put them there as an unconscious cry for help.

Poor eating habits. I had contests with myself to see how long I could go without eating. My goal was to lose weight. I was surprised (and disappointed) when my modeling instructor told me to lose ten pounds. I ended up shedding fifteen. Prior to a modeling job, I would deprive myself of food just to lose an additional pound or two. I would be devastated if I didn't see instant results.

Excessive exercise. This went along with my mission to lose weight. I consistently ran, lifted weights, and did aerobics and toning exercises. I bought a membership to a health club during one of my buying sprees.

Wearing too much makeup. I wore too much eye shadow— probably in an attempt to change my "total being" (after experiencing a period of depression) and to look older. Making myself up made me feel good, another example of poor judgment and inappropriate behavior.

Difficulty completing simple tasks. One year, in a manic phase, I helped my mom to wrap Christmas gifts. The wrapped gifts looked haphazard, similar to my state of mind. I used Disney or Santa Claus wrapping for some of the adult gifts and "adult paper" for some of the kids' presents.

In retrospect, I think it's interesting that I did not mention elevated mood or extreme highs when I listed my manic behaviors and characteristics in my journal. Maybe I didn't consider these feelings to be a liability!

My Symptoms of Depression

Very low self-esteem. I had a modeling job at an upscale clothing store. When I went in for my fitting, the manager said, "You would look great in the pantsuit! It's one of my favorites, and none of the other girls is tiny enough to fit into it." I remember thinking, *Are you talking to me? I feel so fat and ugly.* This occurred when my weight was at its lowest.

Sadness, internal hurt. This sadness never went away. It felt like an elephant was standing on my heart every minute of every day.

Loneliness. I felt isolated and depressed and believed that I had nothing to look forward to in life. At one point I wrote, "I've crawled in my own little hole and I can't get out . . . I'm scared."

Lack of friends. I spent most of the summer of 1978 at home, trying to make sense of what was happening to me. Being so unsure of myself, I wondered if I had any true friends (except for two girls from church who had not been around me as much during my manic episodes). I realized that I wasn't the same person I used to be, and I felt guilty, lonely, and secluded. Sadness engulfed me and I cried frequently. I felt out of touch with the world. My diary describes these feelings in gut-wrenching detail. As I read the entries, I wanted to reach out to that young woman (me) and tell her that everything would be okay. In retrospect, I wished that I could have told her, "You're feeling this way because of a chemical imbalance. It's not something you can control on your own. Let me help you find your way back to peace and happiness."

Overeating at home. I would come home from school, intending to eat a small dish of ice cream. I would end up eating almost the entire half-gallon carton and then feel terrible about myself. This contributed to my feelings of self-loathing.

My mother recalls the following:

> Watching her weight was a trait that Kristin inherited from both her dad and me. We have a tendency to gain a few extra pounds. Healthy eating was number one for me—a challenge, since I'm also a "chocoholic" and love ice cream. When pregnant, I made myself "crave" watermelon, since it was both nutritious and low in calories.
>
> I knew Kristin was eating far too little for a growing teenager. This raised a red flag as I watched her nearly starve herself and then occasionally come home from school and devour all but a fraction of a half-gallon of ice cream straight from the carton. I saw this as yet another example of exaggerated behavior.

Sleeping a lot to escape; napping during the day. Taking naps made me feel safe—especially after school. I tried hard to like school, but I dreaded each day. I felt like an outsider looking in. Sleeping during the day was my haven.

Feeling sometimes that life is not worth living. I will always remember the day I told my mom that I didn't want to live any more. I assured her that I would not act on those feelings because of my religious beliefs and the love I had for my family.

Never buying clothes out of a feeling of worthlessness. I thought that clothes and shoes were too expensive and that I was not worthy to spend money on them. I dressed conservatively and wore very little makeup.

Having nightmares of people killing me. I've blocked out the details of my ongoing nightmares. I do remember that they were vivid and terrifying.

A tendency to overexercise. My tendency to overexercise while I was depressed was different from the tendency to do so when I was manic. During my depressed periods, exercise helped me to experience brief windows of control over my life. It also helped me to lose some of the weight I gained because of food binges. However, I did go through periods when I didn't have the energy to exercise or even accomplish everyday tasks.

My mother had this to say:

Where did my daughter go? Imagine watching your daughter change from a sweet, anxious-to-please, "tattletale" type to a completely different teenager. It started at age thirteen, very slowly and subtly. This type of change is normal, especially in girls. For those who are bipolar, during periods of mania or depression these behaviors are greatly exaggerated.

The combination of my nursing background and observing other family members with bipolar disorder raised a red flag. Sometimes this combination made things even more confusing, because when it's your own child, your feelings prevail over your logic. I felt as vulnerable and as at a loss as any other parent would have.

CONCLUSION

The previous examples serve as a window into the thoughts and feelings I experienced during both extremes of bipolar disorder. I wanted to be aware of these before I stopped taking lithium. My goal was to avoid these behaviors, characteristics, and feelings while I was off medication.

On a day that you're feeling good, you might want to write down your positive attributes. Refer to this list when you (or others) believe that you're going through a manic or depressive phase. Use it to guide you through the hard times. It will also help you to remember your positive qualities.

Julie Fast makes some excellent suggestions in her book, *The Health Cards Treatment System for Bipolar Disorder* (2007). The health cards she has created can supplement your pregnancy journal to help you and your loved ones minimize and manage your bipolar symptoms.

Chapter 4

Off Medication:
Tips for a Smooth Transition

I t is imperative that you talk with your doctors about all medication changes and follow your doctors' recommendations. On January 12, 1991, in preparation for my pregnancy, I started decreasing lithium, as recommended by Dr. Eerdmans. She monitored this process closely.

My therapeutic dose was four 300-milligram (mg) capsules of lithium per day. On January 12, I decreased to three capsules per day. The week of January 19, I went to two capsules per day; the week of January 26, I took only one a day. By February 2, I was off lithium.

On January 14, I wrote the following guidelines to keep my bipolar symptoms in check, and I strove to live by these self-imposed rules:

1. *Concentrate and focus.* This was a priority I tried to apply to all aspects of my life.

2. *Think before talking.*

3. *Don't talk too much—try to resist the pressure to talk.* This was one of my biggest challenges. Self-talk helped me to stay focused. During conversations with others, I trained myself to monitor everything I said *before* talking. I have to admit, however, that I had the hardest time filtering my thoughts when talking with Fred. I concentrated all day, resisting this pressure, and by the time I saw him after work, the floodgates opened. I felt so comfortable with him that I could easily let my thoughts loose.

4. *Increase exercise.* Exercise helped to ease my racing mind by burning off some of my excess energy. It sure made me feel better.

5. *Listen—concentrate and focus on what others are saying.* This was a significant ongoing challenge while I was off lithium. I worked extremely hard to achieve this goal. I was more successful on some days than on others. It helped when I took myself out of the picture and pretended that the person I was talking to was the most important person in the world. I looked directly into people's eyes. I focused and tried to give them the opportunity to finish their sentences before I chimed in.

6. *Be considerate of others.*

7. *Try not to be overly sensitive or defensive about my behaviors or how I react to things.* I had to remember not to be so hard on myself. While off medication, I was unreasonably

critical of how I interacted with others. I questioned many behaviors because I was so afraid of slipping back to the way I used to be prior to my diagnosis. I was determined to prove to myself that I could monitor my behavior.

January 14 [continued]: *From the time I began taking medication, I struggled with the following:*

- *I have to make a conscious effort to let someone finish talking before I contribute to the conversation.*
- *I have to concentrate during church sermons because my mind wanders.*
- *I have to focus when I read.*
- *My mind seems to work overtime—sometimes I think nonstop.*

I wrote in my journal the above four examples to remind myself not to get discouraged when they occurred when I was off lithium—after all, they were common when I was *on* medication! I wanted to have realistic expectations and avoid setting myself up for disappointment. I had to remind myself that I was not "superwoman"—even when on lithium.

I suggest that you write down some of the behaviors that are common to you now, prior to discontinuing or reducing your medication. It will help you to keep them in perspective. Talk to your support team and refer to your journal often to help guide you and keep you on track.

Writing down the list of manic and depressive behaviors I lived with in the past reminded me that these behaviors and symptoms were due to my bipolar condition, not to me. I referred to this information often, from the preconception phase to postpartum. It was concrete evidence that my unpredictable behavior was caused by a chemical imbalance and that I couldn't rely on lithium for self-control. My intent was to refer to this journal entry to increase awareness of the bipolar symptoms that I knew were right around the corner.

I was petrified before stopping lithium. My seven guidelines helped me to regain some of the control that I knew I was going to lose. (Chapter 10 elaborates on the importance of understanding how a person's prefrontal lobe functions. It's a fascinating concept and will prove to be helpful for those who stop their medication.) As I was weaning myself off lithium, I wrote in my journal nearly every day. Once I wrote something down, it freed up my mind—I didn't have to remember it anymore.

Having a destination for your thoughts is especially important before you go to sleep at night. That's why I usually wrote in my journal in the evening. I was more wound up at that time. Sometimes I wrote brief summaries, and at other times my thoughts came at me faster than I could write them down. The need to record them was unyielding and addicting. I would write until Fred said, "Kristin, it's time to finish up and put your journal away."

Write in your journal at different times of the day to see what works best for you. It might be most helpful to write in the morning, before starting your day. Give yourself a pep talk in your journal. Use it to help define each day and to navigate through this transition. Your journal is also an excellent way to manage apprehension, fear, and frustration. The important thing is to write in it regularly.

My mother had this to say about keeping a journal:

Kristin's grandma, my mom, kept a daily diary from ages fourteen to eighty-four. I still have my five-year diaries written from ages fourteen to twenty-four. So it was natural for Kristin to be a faithful diary writer. Again, the red flag of exaggerated behavior popped up when I'd find pages of her writings, usually stuffed under her bed. A light came on much later, when I realized this was a well-developed coping skill.

January 21: On January 19, I decreased my lithium dose to two tablets a day. The week of January 11, I felt great taking three a day. I didn't even notice that much difference. Today is my third day taking only two tablets a day.

I really noticed a difference in my "sharpness" while talking on the phone to potential exhibitors. It seems as if my mind knows how to respond to their objections, but when I verbalize it, my response is not as crisp. Maybe I'm overreacting, but it seems as if I'm having a little bit of trouble expressing (verbally) what I'm thinking.

Based on the observations noted in my next journal entry, I think I was overreacting.

Shortly after beginning my job as a marketing consultant, I made it a point to get to know my coworker. She was smart, levelheaded, and honest. I told her about my situation because I trusted her and knew the importance of occasionally relying on her judgment. Examples will follow in this chapter. She was supportive and understanding.

Prior to your medication changes, identify trusted people in your life that you can depend on to share their judgment. Try to be responsive and respectful of their feedback. They can help you monitor your behavior while giving you an outlet for second-guessing yourself. You don't have to do this alone.

January 22: I feel great today. I had breakfast with my coworker and lunch with a good friend, and neither one noticed any change in me.

I asked for feedback because I trusted and respected them. I was conscientious and guarded every time I had a conversation with anyone (except Fred—poor Fred). It surprised me when no change was apparent. I'm certain that they didn't understand how much I had to concentrate to give this impression.

Talking to people who were aware of our goal to start a family was comforting. It was helpful to discuss how much I wanted to get pregnant, the normal fears about having a baby, and how this change would affect our lives. In addition, it was therapeutic to communicate my fear of going off lithium. Verbalizing these concerns felt good. I didn't even feel the pressure to talk during our conversations.

I even felt competent driving a car. If anything, I was more cautious. Once again, heightened awareness helped me to overcome my tendency to drive too fast while my lithium was being *was probably due to the stress created by my pharmaceutical position and my anxiety about our uncertain future.*

I would not have told my manager about having bipolar disorder if it had been imperative for me to keep my job. I could afford to tell her because we were not dependent on my part-time income.

February 1: I have felt 100 percent all week. Tomorrow I'll be off lithium. Wednesday night and Thursday were tough at Grandpa's funeral. I will miss him. Visiting with my relatives and immediate family was fun. I think that was the "true test" in terms of how I'm doing off lithium. I felt comfortable talking with them about how things are going, and about my new job.

However, I was very conscious of how I communicated with everyone. It was a challenge for me to filter everything I said. Deciding what to say and what to keep to myself took concentration. If I was around people who didn't know I was bipolar, I had a tendency to put my guard up. I tried to make sure my behavior was "appropriate."

February 1 [continued]: Tonight Fred and I are going out to dinner to celebrate his birthday. I'm really looking forward to a night out together! [In the margin I wrote:] *Work continues to go well. I contacted approximately forty people today by phone about exhibiting* [promoting their business] *in the trade show.*

Self-discipline enabled me to accomplish whatever goal I set for the day.

Increased productivity is one of the many benefits of being bipolar. My drive to succeed enabled me to work efficiently. However,

reduced. I was a safe and conscientious driver when I was off medication.

Medication changes may make you overly critical and sensitive. Try not to question yourself. Write your progress down, as I did.

Each day can feel like a new experience as you make medication adjustments. Don't overanalyze how you feel. Write down your thoughts and move on. I frequently read previous journal entries because they helped me to realize how fast my perceptions and emotions changed. During difficult times, they were proof that "this too shall pass."

January 22 [continued]: I was proud of myself at the mall today. The only thing I bought was barrettes. I didn't even have the urge to buy anything else. If I could pinpoint any changes that I'm experiencing today, the only one that comes to mind is that I feel elated.

I vividly remember thinking that I might not be able to control an urge to buy clothes—I love to buy clothes and shoes. I knew I would be able to rationalize any purchase. My increased awareness about spending money frivolously was helpful.

January 28: Yesterday, Fred and I went to a Super Bowl party. All of Fred's softball buddies and their spouses were there. Fred told me last night that he hasn't noticed any difference in my behavior.

This party was the first social situation I attended in which I felt outside my comfort zone. I didn't see these friends often, and I felt as if I had a message tattooed on my forehead that said, "I am bipolar, and I am almost off my medication." I wanted them to know I was trying my hardest to act appropriately. I couldn't even ask anyone if I was acting normal because no one knew I was bipolar. I just wasn't ready to tell them.

When people asked me about my job, I couldn't explain why I left my pharmaceutical career to work part time as a marketing consultant for a trade show. I wanted to shout from the rooftop that Fred and I were planning on having a baby. My guard was up the entire evening; I was self-conscious. I realized that there were going to be numerous social occasions like this when I would have to conceal what was really going on. Because of this, I knew that it was necessary for me to train myself to feel comfortable and confident in social situations.

Fred noted the following:

I did not see a significant change in Kristin's behavior as she reduced her lithium. She was very aware of her behavior before she was diagnosed. It was important to maintain the consistency in her daily routine while she was off the medication.

January 28 [continued]: *Sunday morning, I found out my Grandpa McCulloch passed away. I cried tears full of mixed emotions. I do realize he's not in discomfort or pain any longer. He is now in heaven with my grandma.*

January 29: I'm still feeling great. I had lunch with my friend who is a clinical nurse specialist at an area hospital. I'm happy because I have not felt pressure to talk—my mind is not racing! She told me if anything, I seem more relaxed—less stressed out.

While I was a medical center representative, our rela[tionship] evolved into a personal one, and I felt comfortable upda[ting] about my plans to have a baby. Sharing our exciting new[s with] someone who supported me and seemed to understand th[e chal]lenges I was facing was liberating.

I had not talked about my bipolar condition with many p[eople] who were not close friends—most of my relatives didn't [even] know I was bipolar. I was afraid of their reaction. I felt so g[ood] telling her about the challenges I faced as a bipolar—she w[as] interested but not uncomfortable or judgmental.

Deciding to have a baby is exciting. Determining with whom to share your news—at least the chemical imbalance aspect— can be tough. I was selective about whom I would tell that I was bipolar. Here are two general guidelines you should consider: Share with people you trust and who will be supportive. Avoid telling those who might discriminate against you. For example, if you are working, use discretion if you decide to tell your boss or coworkers. Reconsider if you have anything to lose. It's a shame to have to consider discrimination, but it's best to be cautious.

January 29 [continued]: *My trade show manager told me she hasn't noticed any difference in my behavior and is impressed with my performance.* [I summarized my situation to her once I proved I could effectively do my job. I was encouraged by her feedback because in four days I would be off lithium.] *She told me that when I first interviewed with her, I almost didn't get the job because I was so intense and it seemed that I was under a lot of stress. That* it was an ongoing challenge to strike a balance. Exaggerated behavior is a common characteristic of bipolar disorder.

February 15: I have consistently felt great! Better than I've felt since I can remember. My job situation is improving. I have the following system for selling booth/exhibit space: (1) Contact decision maker or leave a message that I am sending information on _____ day and will follow up on _____ or _____ day. (2) Send information. (3) Follow up on the day(s) specified in the first call.

I was more balanced when I had a detailed plan of action. Uncertainty created anxiety for me.

February 15 [continued]: Friday, February 8, was the turning point for the success I've been having selling exhibit space. I'm excited because now I can contact (and have been contacting all week) all my "on the fence" accounts (as well as accounts that have already said no) and sell them on the benefits of attending the trade show in March. Once they attend, most of them will be sold on securing an exhibit for our next trade show.

I am very frustrated with my manager. At my request, she gives me specific dates when she'll complete something that she has promised my coworker and me. When the target date approaches, she gives me excuses as to why it's not done. In the meantime, I've contacted my accounts and have a specific date to follow up, based on the fact that they should receive their information and have time to review it by the time I call them.

My manager told me that I shouldn't give specific dates when I'm sending information to them. She said I should tell them I'd send the information soon (whatever that means). Today on the phone I told her exactly how I felt about her not following up on her commitment. I was very tough on her.

I get frustrated when people tell me they are going to do something and don't follow through with it. This attribute was intensified while I was off medication. I can't blame my bipolar symptoms for the candid conversation I had with my manager. I wasn't rude; I simply summarized how I felt. Talking with my coworker about how I handled it was validating. She felt the same way.

February 15 [continued]: Despite the fact she is keeping me from doing (performing) my best, I still feel very good about me. I'm trying to keep this in perspective. I'm doing the best job I can.

February 20: I sure wish I was doing as well as I was on February 15 and prior to that date. (I felt great—very relaxed.) I'm accomplishing a lot, but I've been working a forty-hour week for the last two weeks and haven't made much money.

On the positive side, I know I'll sell several exhibitor booths by May. My goal is to sell between fifty and seventy-five booths. If I do that, I'll gross about _____. That's really not much money for four and a half months of hard work— January 1 to May 15.

The real kicker is that Monday, Tuesday, and Wednesday of this week I've felt uptight and stressed out. For the past two weeks especially, I've been working extremely hard and long hours. It's not worth it because I'm not making much money.

At this point, I knew I needed to rearrange my thinking, so I developed the following action plan: *Put this job into perspective. Set daily goals that are attainable without getting stressed out. Work on calling a specified number of accounts, then stop.*

Enjoy the benefits of this part-time, flexible job. I set the following limits on myself:

- *Stop working by 5:00–6:00 P.M. (including paperwork).*
- *Don't work evenings.* I know this is repeating myself, but I must have thought it was necessary when I made the list. Manic phases can do that to you.
- *Don't think about work so much.*
- *Don't think I have to give 100 percent in order for this show to be a success.* At the same time, I was determined to make this year's show a success. I believed that I owed it to my clients because they trusted me when I sold them on the benefits of exhibiting.

Notice how the last item seems to contain a contradiction. My goals frequently contradicted my behavior. I documented them because I realized that it was best for me to keep track of them. Nevertheless, bipolar disorder seemed to conquer my rational thinking.

I tried hard to control my overdrive, but sometimes my stress level would be reduced if I worked longer hours rather than thinking about what needed to get done.

February 20 [continued]: *I want them to feel as if they're getting their money's worth. Keep in mind that all these goals can be accomplished even if I "slow down" and work smarter. I'll continue to work hard but work fewer hours. I'm committed to following these goals. I've got to slow down for my health and for Fred.*

It seemed as if the real me and my bipolar symptoms were constantly at war with each other. Fred made the following observation:

> I knew Kristin had been working too many hours. This was supposed to be a part-time job—less stress, fewer hours. However, Kristin has always put customers first and is extremely motivated to work hard. She knew she needed to slow down and let her manager help with the details of the trade show; however, I wasn't sure she was capable of doing this.

Miklowitz (2002) reports that, in his experience:

> . . . people with bipolar disorder are able to benefit from hypomania in the work setting only if they are able to harness it. Harnessing hypomania includes learning to recognize when you are moving or speaking too fast, setting limits on yourself when work starts to make you overly goal-driven, trying to accomplish only one task at a time, accepting feedback from others about how you are coming across, and backing off when people seem to be reacting to your intensity. It may indeed be possible to translate your increased energy into work productivity, but also be aware of when you need to slow down and take a break. (p. 277)

It's as if he wrote this just for me!

February 21: I didn't sleep well on Monday, Tuesday, or Wednesday of this week. My mind doesn't stop thinking. I worry about the dumbest things. Example: owning a car wash and not having enough water to run it—silly things. I would love to be able to sleep without being interrupted by my thoughts.

February 26: My mission lately has been to set reasonable daily goals for work. I continue to work about forty hours a week because I want to contact as many businesses as possible prior to March 7. We're leaving to ski in Vail, Colorado, and won't return until March 17. The trade show is coming up soon.

I have not had a difficult time sleeping since February 21. My mind isn't racing at night as much as it was before. [Writing in my journal before going to bed helped me compartmentalize my racing thoughts.]

I will not let this job get the best of me. I keep reminding myself to keep it in perspective. No amount of money can justify feeling so stressed. I'll continue to set realistic daily goals. I know that I'm putting all my effort into this job—that's all I have control over. Working from 8:30 A.M. until 5:00 or 6:00 P.M. should be enough.

Of course it was enough—it was a part-time job.

As I mentioned earlier, increased productivity can be a positive aspect of bipolar disorder. For me, at times, it ignited my manic symptoms. What types of things ignite your manic or depressive symptoms? Identify the people in your life who can help you maintain a balance. Talk to them before your medication changes to establish your expectations. Recording your activities and the amount of time you spend on them in your journal will help you to keep track of your actions.

February 26 [continued]: *Although I'm working excessively, I know I should not feel compelled to work more (this is how I do feel).*

My work is directly related to the success of the show. That statement is somewhat true, but I have to remember that I'm only one person and I shouldn't feel as if the success of this show is dependent on me putting all my time and energy into it.

Although I had written an action plan in my journal just six days earlier, I felt the need to reel myself in once again. I used the following list as a guideline to help keep me on track. At times, this felt like a constant battle. This was my list of priorities:

1. *Read the Bible.*
2. *Spend time with Fred.*
3. *Work out.*
4. *Spend time with my friends and family.*
5. *Attend to bills and personal matters, such as keeping my office in order.*

"Kristin used her list of priorities to help manage each day," Fred noted. "She was determined to regulate her actions. This list helped her keep most things in perspective, but she couldn't see that she was still working too many hours."

My mom added the following:

During the time she was without lithium, I was so grateful that Kristin had a written plan as well as a supportive husband, doctors, and friends. Nurse Mom wished we lived closer than a two-hour drive. Frequent phone conversations, visits, and lots of prayers helped me cope.

I talked with my coworker regularly to get feedback about my behavior. It was important for me to make sure I acted appropriately. My coworker was the mirror to help me see myself professionally. It's beneficial to have trustworthy people from various aspects of your life who can provide you with a way to see yourself realistically during this challenging and unpredictable time.

For example, I called my coworker periodically after talking to a prospect over the phone or in person. I would summarize the conversation and ask her if I communicated effectively and appropriately. I mentioned that my mind was racing and so I wasn't sure if I was making sense. I tried so hard to manage my thoughts, and I wasn't certain if they were deceiving me.

My coworker usually told me that she would have handled the conversation in a similar way. She validated me and gave me the confidence to trust that I had presented my thoughts rationally and succinctly, even though my mind was unsettled and fragmented.

If you don't have the luxury of using a coworker to help you see yourself during medication changes, rely on a trusted friend, family member, or bipolar support group member to provide you with insight about work. Prior to making medication changes, ask people you trust to help you monitor your manic and depressive phases. Provide them with guidelines. Choose those who are diplomatic and caring. Give them permission to share accurate feedback with you and your partner. Their input could help you to get the proper and necessary assistance. Your selected supporters, however, should keep the following information in mind.

Miklowitz (2002) writes the following about many of the challenges faced by anyone who has an illness.

Close relatives should be involved in the care of any person with a chronic illness, whether it is a psychiatric disorder or a traditional medical disorder like heart disease. We know from research in health psychology that people who have the best healthcare practices tend to engage family members in changing their unwanted habits. For example, their family members encourage them to eat healthy foods, avoid smoking, or get exercise. However, involving others is a double-edged sword: Accepting the help or oversight of another person will probably generate a certain amount of psychological distress in you (Lewis & Rook, 1999).

What is this distress about? Most people resent the idea of having others—particularly their close relatives—in a position of authority when they start to become ill. In the extreme, it can feel like agreeing to have someone else take away your independence. These are understandable reactions shared by people with many other medical illnesses. For example, people with insulin-dependent diabetes dislike the idea that someone else might have to inject them if they go into shock. People with high blood pressure or cardiovascular diseases dislike the idea that a spouse might monitor their food or salt intake.

People with bipolar disorder seem especially prone to feeling this way. I have heard the statement "I hate the idea of giving up control to anyone" from many clients, whether the control is being given up to a lover, a spouse, a doctor, or (especially) a parent. I think there are several reasons [that] the issue of control is so salient to people with bipolar disorder. First, when you experience the internal feelings of chaos that mood fluctuations cause, it can become especially important to feel [as if] you're at least in control of your outside world. Second, the feelings of confidence and power associated with the early and later stages of mania make you especially prone to rejecting the advice, opinions, or direct help of others. Third, many people with bipolar disorder have had bad experiences in the past when others—however well-intentioned— tried to exert control over them during emergencies. (p. 188)

March 2: My job is still putting tons of pressure on me because I continue to work too many hours for so little money. The long hours began the week ending February 15—forty-two hours; then February 22, forty-three hours, and March 1, forty-five hours. These hours include fifteen minutes one way to work (I don't include my travel time home), all office time in my home (including paper-work), hours at the downtown office, and lunch breaks. For the past three weeks, I have taken no breaks in the morning or afternoon.

On February 28 and March 1, I had a glass of wine in the evening. Both nights I slept soundly. Now here's my rationale: I should not have to drink a glass of wine before going to bed to help me get a restful sleep.

Here is another interesting point: I find it necessary to limit myself on the amount of work I do. Example: It's 2:00 P.M. today (Saturday). My goal is to organize my office and complete my personal business (bills and miscellaneous) for a while this afternoon. I told myself I can't do any trade show paperwork—even though part of me wants to work on it before I start my personal paperwork. I haven't taken time for personal paperwork in weeks. [I didn't like being disorganized.] *I shouldn't have to put limits on myself about "not working today"—it's Saturday. I do plan on working on the showcase tomorrow.*

If I were like most people with a part-time job, I'd close my office door and wouldn't work at home. Keeping in mind that we're going to Colorado Thursday, I know if I don't do my trade show paperwork tomorrow, I'll be more vulnerable to stress on Monday.

Next week will be incredibly busy for me because I plan on preparing several prospective client lists and organizing trade show information packets to be mailed while I'm in Colorado. The work I accomplish Monday–Thursday will determine how much gets done when I'm on vacation. (My manager told me that if I give her this information before leaving, including addresses of each business, she'll have the labels typed and the packets of showcase literature assembled.)

I will put more effort into not feeling overwhelmed about everything that needs to be done instead of dwelling on it. More important, I should not be thinking about it now; it's time to enjoy the weekend—after I do my personal paperwork, of course.

March 3: Yesterday afternoon, I ended up cleaning the house and preparing for a small dinner party for friends. They came over for quiche last night. It's 4:00 P.M. and I'm just starting my personal paperwork. I sure do hate doing paperwork!

March 7: Thursday, 10:30 P.M. We left for Colorado. We're driving a minivan straight through [my parents were with us].

March 8: Friday morning: I had no problem sleeping in the van.

March 14: We're all having a phenomenal time out here skiing. I feel fantastic! I have not thought about work at all. Interesting point—when I feel really good (not stressed out, less pressure to talk), I don't need to write in this journal. On the days that I feel stressed out, writing my feelings in my journal is an outlet.

Enough said. One more thing: This vacation has made me put my work into perspective. I've been putting in way too many hours. Next week my goal is to have control of the number of hours that I work and think about work.

Even on the days that I was feeling good, it was difficult for me to succinctly write what was on my mind. I often felt the need to add one more thought or goal. I did this because having a "parking place" for my rapid thoughts was soothing. I also hoped that reviewing my seemingly levelheaded intentions would help to keep me on track.

Fred said the following:

Our ski trip to Colorado couldn't have come at a better time. The decision to have a baby and the associated medical concerns for Kristin were stressful for both of us. We were traveling with her parents and would see her two brothers who were living in Colorado at the time. I think being close to her family at this time was comforting for Kristin. Being away from work, the beautiful scenery, and skiing in the mountain air made her stress melt away.

We're at It Again:
Going Off Medication for Our Second Baby

I frequently referred to my pregnancy journal for guidance and support as I prepared to go off lithium a second time. The one difference is that after I resumed lithium following Katherine's birth (my first pregnancy), Dr. Eerdmans decreased my maintenance dose to three 300-mg capsules a day instead of four. In preparation for my second pregnancy, she suggested the following plan to discontinue lithium:

November 23–30: two capsules a day
December 1–7: one capsule a day
December 8: no lithium

Lithium would then be out of my system by around December 19.

Following a documented action plan and my previous journal entries helped me to focus on our goal of having a second baby. Again, ongoing communication with my psychiatrist was an important part of the process. Even though I anticipated experiencing temporary manic and depressive episodes, at times they seemed so permanent.

In this next journal entry I describe a manic episode.

January 14, 1994, A.M.: My mind is racing so fast I don't know where to begin. I feel as if I'm on a train (on the outside hanging on, not in a comfortable seat inside) going really fast. I wish I could jump off to slow myself down.

When I'm having a conversation with someone, it's hard for me to follow them at their slow pace. My mind processes the information at such a fast rate. I feel as if I know where their conversation is going before they verbalize it to me.

I know this will pass. I have a feeling I'll see improvement (experience peace of mind again) once I get pregnant. Once I'm pregnant I will be able to see the light at the end of the tunnel (I'll be closer to being able to go back on lithium).

Two minutes later—I feel so isolated. Not many people understand what I'm going through. I just caught myself going through my phone book looking for someone I could call to talk with—someone who understands bipolar disorder. I wish I had someone to talk to—someone who can identify with how I'm feeling.

I vividly remember this experience. I felt so desperate and hopeless. I ended up not calling anyone to share how I was feeling. I truly thought no one could understand or relate to my racing mind or my feelings of isolation.

January 14, P.M.: I feel a lot better now. Fred just got home and I'm looking forward to a nice, quiet weekend with him and Katherine.

As you can see, there were days when I felt as if I were on an emotional roller coaster. These January 14 excerpts are an excellent example of temporary bipolar phases. I referred to them when I needed to be reminded that these agonizing feelings were not permanent. It helped me to keep things in perspective.

SUMMARY

Going off medication or making medication changes is an important step prior to conception. The following techniques can help in this process:

- Document bipolar symptoms that you have experienced.

- Review these bipolar symptoms to increase your awareness.

- Refer to this list while you're off medication (or if there are changes in medication).

- Remember that these symptoms are caused by your chemical imbalance—they are *temporary*; they don't define you.

- Talk with your psychiatrist or doctor about a plan for medication changes.

- Write the plan down and follow it.

- Know when it's safe to try to conceive.

- Use your partner, psychiatrist or doctor, trusted friend, relative, or coworker as a mirror to see yourself.

- Join a bipolar support group.

- Write in your journal to
    - ✓ monitor your symptoms and progress;
    - ✓ communicate your thoughts and feelings;
    - ✓ use as a coach and advocate;
    - ✓ compartmentalize racing thoughts;

✓ provide a picture of overall behavior;

✓ keep your priorities in perspective;

✓ provide an outlet for bipolar phases.

• Review the material in your inspirational shoe box
(see Chapter 3).

Doctor's Note

BY JAY CARTER, PsyD, DABPS

If you are planning to become pregnant, there are two significant ways to prevent a bipolar episode from occurring: Get enough sleep and maintain a routine.

Circadian rhythm changes should be avoided. I would discourage going to Europe while off medication because the time zone changes can set off an episode. A six- to eight-hour difference is very risky, and also the hustle-bustle of Europe is stressful. Go to the Poconos and rest up, instead!

Most people who have the bipolar genes think out of the box, but they need a BOX TO THINK OUT OF. Have a daily routine.

Journaling is a great way to "see yourself." It makes you re-enter your prefrontal lobe. It reminds you of the bigger picture so you don't get caught up in the racing details. It reminds you of your purpose and what is most important.

Even if you don't feel like journaling, make yourself feel like journaling.

And, of course, avoid stress at all costs.

Chapter 5

My First Pregnancy

Fred and I were mentally and emotionally ready for me to get pregnant. I was conscious of and looking for changes in my body that revealed signs of a new life inside me. I felt confident that once I got pregnant, the end result was within reach. I knew that within a year of that happy day, we would have a baby, and I would be able to resume taking lithium. Yay! That gave me peace of mind.

March 24, 1991: I felt a wave of nausea the morning of March 17, on our way home from Vail, Colorado. My period wasn't due until March 19, and this was a positive sign. The morning of March 21, I had a pregnancy test at a clinic. It was faintly positive. I looked at the test again at 2:30, and the positive sign was darker. I needed to be sure before I told Fred, so later that afternoon I went back to the clinic for another test. This one was definitely POSITIVE!

At first, I was more shocked than excited. When I told Fred, the first thing he said was "Are you sure?" I told him about the pregnancy test, and I can still see his smile. Today, just for fun, we bought a home pregnancy test and saw the results together. The positive sign showed up immediately. Fred is more convinced now. We're both so excited! The high we feel is incredible.

Fred said the following:

> When Kristin told me she was pregnant, I was so surprised, almost shocked that it happened so fast. I knew she had been keeping track of when she ovulated, but still, I thought it would take much longer. I was ecstatic about being a father! I was also happy for Kristin for two reasons. One, I knew how much she wanted to be a mom, and two, it would be a minimum amount of time for her to be off lithium.

Once I knew I was pregnant, I bought the book *What to Expect When You're Expecting,* by Heidi Murkoff, Arlene Eisenberg, and Sandee Hathaway. It was my primary reference and road map throughout my pregnancy. This pregnancy guide provides pertinent information and addresses concerns from the planning stage through postpartum. I especially enjoyed the question-and-answer sections and insightful facts on what to expect during each month of a pregnancy. My pregnancy was a month-to-month journey. My goal was to enjoy each phase. I read the chapters in order, concentrating on one month at a time. I tried not to read ahead. It was a treat to read about what was in store for me during the month I was experiencing it.

March 30: I've been making a conscious effort to reduce my work hours to twenty to thirty per week. I have to reduce my stress level. The week ending March 22, I worked twenty-six hours, and the week ending March 29, I worked twenty-one hours. I think I have my work schedule under control. Now I have a good reason to limit my hours.

Fred added the following:

I noticed a change in Kristin after she reduced her workload. Working about thirty hours per week gave her more time to relax and think about being a mom. Just the sheer joy of having our first baby made the days seem much less demanding.

I made the decision not to use my pregnancy as an excuse to gain excessive weight and continued to exercise about five days a week. It's worth mentioning again that exercise has additional benefits for women who are both bipolar and pregnant. It can help you to get through potential manic and depressive episodes. For example, exercise can help you to regain temporary control of your life when you feel as if your mind won't stop racing or when you're sad or feeling isolated.

Prior to beginning an exercise program, it's important to get approval from your physician. The March of Dimes article "Fitness for Two" (www.marchofdimes.com) answers the question "Does pregnancy change how a woman's body responds to physical activity?" It explains as follows:

During pregnancy, a woman's body changes in a number of ways that alter her response to exercise. For example, a pregnant woman's tolerance for strenuous exercise decreases as pregnancy progresses. Pregnant women require more oxygen than nonpregnant women, even at rest. As pregnancy progresses, women have to work harder to breathe because the enlarging uterus crowds the diaphragm (the large muscle separating the chest and abdomen). These changes mean that there is less oxygen available for use during exercise, making it easier to become out of breath. . . .

Pregnant women should take steps to avoid overheating, especially during the first trimester, because during this time a sustained body temperature of 102.5° F or higher may increase the risk of certain birth defects of the brain and spine. However, studies have not shown any increase in these or other birth defects among babies of women who exercise vigorously during pregnancy.

Pregnancy alters a woman's sense of balance. The enlarging uterus and breasts shift her center of gravity. High hormone levels make her connective tissues more lax and her joints may be more susceptible to injury. All of these changes determine the types of exercises that are safest for pregnant women. . . .

What types of exercise are best during pregnancy? Most pregnant women can continue their pre-pregnancy exercise programs, though they may need to modify some activities or decrease the intensity of workouts as pregnancy progresses. For example, a jogger who quickly becomes fatigued or breathless may switch to brisk walking.

A pregnant woman should stop exercising immediately if she experiences symptoms such as vaginal bleeding, dizziness, shortness of breath, headache, chest pain, muscle weakness, calf pain or swelling, uterine contractions, or amniotic fluid leakage.

Women who perform non-weight-bearing activities, such as cycling or swimming, are more likely to be able to continue exercising at high intensity through the third trimester than women who perform weight-bearing exercises, such as jogging or aerobic dancing. Non-weight-bearing activities appear to decrease the risk of injury, though bicycle riders may want to switch to a stationary bicycle, because it may be more difficult to maintain balance as pregnancy proceeds. Women who lift weights can safely continue to train with light weights (about 5 to 10 pounds) but should probably avoid lifting heavier weights or lifting weights while lying flat on their backs. If a pregnant woman is just starting an exercise program (with her health care provider's okay), walking, swimming, and cycling on a stationary bicycle are activities that are usually safe. (pp. 2–3)

The licensed physical therapist I went to while pregnant and after delivery led a prenatal and postpartum exercise program sponsored by her company. An exercise specialist, with a background in exercise physiology, and a certified occupational therapy assistant led the class as well. Contact physical therapy facilities in your area to see if they offer prenatal and postpartum exercise programs.

Check with a hospital in your area for pregnancy and parenting classes. They are designed to help you prepare for your baby's birth and to learn about the infant care. Another option is a hospital birthing center, known for warm, personal one-on-one care. If you need advanced medical care, it's usually available there.

Keep in mind that women who have bipolar disorder and are pregnant have all these issues to consider in addition to managing their symptoms. I continued to write in my pregnancy journal during my pregnancy and postpartum to help me manage and cope with my unpredictable mood swings. My journal was also an outlet for the uncomfortable and exciting body changes I felt because of my growing baby. It was helpful to look back and remind myself that all my discomforts were temporary. It helped me to realize I could get past each one. I also liked to review the exciting moments during the pregnancy that I'll treasure forever. You think you'll always remember the details, but writing them down evokes clearer memories.

April 4: I had my six- to eight-week checkup (prenatal education) with the nurse. She gave me a helpful tip to decrease the terrible nausea I've been experiencing. She recommended that I should avoid drinking liquids with meals. It's best to wait forty-five minutes after a meal before drinking anything. She also told me to eat saltine crackers before I get out of bed in the morning. I carry them with me everywhere I go. I started following this advice, and I felt much better. (I still get nauseous, but it's not as bad.) Prior to April 4, I felt nauseous twenty-four hours a day. It's discouraging to feel nauseous in the middle of the night when I get up to use the bathroom.

I felt like I couldn't escape it.

April 17: Fred and I were in Boston from April 13–17. He ran in the Boston Marathon. I felt sick the entire time. The night before he ran, we went out for pasta dinner, and the smell of Parmesan cheese made me feel worse. [I became a true believer that when you're pregnant, your sense of smell is heightened. Some of my favorite foods smelled like rotten eggs.] We went to Cheers for lunch, and the only thing I could eat was tomato soup and crackers.

April 29: I've been feeling better since April 25, although some days I still feel nauseous. Prior to the 25th, I could only eat crackers, yogurt, cottage cheese, and soup. It's great to be able to eat different foods again (I still can't eat sandwiches).

I recorded in detail what I ate because it was encouraging to me that my tolerance for food increased as my nausea decreased. Those who know me well know that when I'm healthy, I start looking forward to my next meal shortly after I finish the previous one. Eating is one of my favorite things!

May 5: My nausea is the worst from dinnertime until I go to bed. Today I had half a turkey and cheese sandwich for the first time since becoming pregnant. It was OK because I ate it without toasting the bread. That's strange, because I normally love toasted bread.

I spoke too soon—I guess "feeling better" means that I'm not nauseous twenty-four hours a day. It is getting better, though. My appetite is increasing as well.

May 24: I can see a steady change in my weight. I have been recording my weight almost daily since my first month. [I admit that's obsessive, but it helped me to reach my goal of gaining no more than 30 pounds.] On May 22, I bought maternity shorts and pants.

It was fun trying on clothes at the maternity store. I put a pregnancy pillow under one of the shirts I bought to see what I would look like once the baby became bigger. I felt kind of silly, but at the same time my anticipation and excitement were heightened.

May 24 [continued]: *Today I had my first checkup with Dr. Hiemenga* [my ob-gyn]. *I'm in my thirteenth week. (I had an appointment on May 16, but I wasn't able to see her because she was delivering a baby.) I heard our baby's heartbeat! It was so exciting— tears came to my eyes.*

Early on I learned that I needed to be flexible and patient for all prenatal appointments. During future appointments I had to remind myself that sometime in the near future, it could be the delivery of *my* baby that keeps Dr. Hiemenga from being available or on time for someone else.

During this first appointment with Dr. Hiemenga, I started recording the following information: the date of each prenatal appointment, the pregnancy week I was in, my weight, the baby's heart rate, and my blood pressure. I continued recording this information through my final prenatal visit. I liked to keep track of these facts because it gave me a sense of control and active participation during my pregnancy.

Everything that I could do to regain control while off lithium was helpful. Before your medication changes, think of ways you can increase control of your life during this uncertain time.

Reviewing the ongoing progress of your baby's development also adds to your involvement throughout the pregnancy. There are several ways to do this.

Your Pregnancy Journal Week by Week by Glade B. Curtis and Judith Schuler (2002) can be used to record this information for each prenatal appointment. Additional topics include your medical history, recording "firsts" during your pregnancy, childbirth education classes, a labor and delivery summary, your experience with the baby in the hospital, and the after-delivery experience. I would have loved to have had a book like this to help me organize this important information. (It was published after my pregnancies.) It also serves as a keepsake of your pregnancy.

Another organizer is *What to Expect Pregnancy Journal & Organizer,* by Heidi Murkoff with Sharon Mazel (2007). Pick the method that appeals to you.

June 18: Memorial Day weekend I noticed that I'm consistently starting to feel better. I don't even have to eat saltine crackers in the morning before getting out of bed. Standing up for long periods of time at church makes me dizzy and sick to my stomach. On occasion I get pains in my stomach. It feels like knives—it's probably ligaments stretching. Every once in a while, I feel Roscoe kicking [it's embarrassing to admit this, but Fred and I referred to our unborn baby as Roscoe instead of calling him or her "baby" all the time]. *I have to put my hand on my stomach and feel for the movement.*

June 27 [eighteen weeks]: *Last night I definitely felt Roscoe kicking! Early this morning, I felt him for a while, too. It's much stronger than before. I still have to put my hand on my stomach to feel him. I continue to feel great.*

July 4: Roscoe's kicking is getting stronger. This weekend, Fred felt a strong kick. I continue to feel good, although I get tired when I'm not active.

We were both elated. Feeling our baby's movement inside me is something we'll always remember—it's magical.

July 16: I had an ultrasound today [almost twenty-one weeks]. *Fred and I do not want to know if Roscoe is a boy or girl. Roscoe was in the fetal position the entire forty-five minutes. The technician was still able take the pictures needed, including Roscoe's heart and placenta.*

Fred came with me to the appointment. It was incredible seeing our baby—especially when he moved around. Fred heard Roscoe's heartbeat, too. Later in the day, the nurse called and told me everything about the ultrasound looked good. We're so excited!

We wanted to be surprised about the sex of our child. I compared it to eating Cracker Jacks as a kid and waiting to discover the prize at the bottom of the box. We wanted the anticipation and surprise to follow us during the duration of our pregnancy. I will always treasure the first pictures of our baby.

Fred noted the following:

The ultrasound was a very rewarding experience. To see a picture of your unborn child is quite miraculous! I took two of the pictures to work to show my coworkers and kept them on my desk. Hearing our baby's heartbeat was further confirmation that parenthood was on the way. I encourage any father-to-be to take the time, if possible, to go to an ultrasound or routine appointment. It will be an unforgettable experience.

July 31: I've felt really good since June. The first three months of pregnancy I was nauseous practically twenty-four hours a day. August 2 is my last day as a marketing consultant. I gave my two-week notice July 18.

I was an independent contractor, paid by commission, so I felt comfortable wrapping up the project I was working on to pursue another opportunity that better suited my needs.

I have always been good at prospecting and setting up appointments. Within days, my dad hired me to schedule appointments for him here in town. I prepared a script (talk track) and referred to it during each call. I'd been working in sales for so long that when I learned the prospective client was not interested in meeting with my dad, I understood that he or she was rejecting his service or product, not me personally. I was fully aware that it was a numbers game. The more no's I heard, the closer I was to hearing a yes. I had control of my schedule and the number of hours that I chose to work. It worked out really well.

Initially, I chose to limit my hours to four per day because I almost always overextended myself. The commitment to curb my drive was helpful but not effective. Less than three weeks after I began working with my dad, I jumped at the opportunity to increase my productivity. This is another example of my exaggerated behavior.

Even as I was scheduling appointments for my dad, I also felt the need to take on more responsibility. I loved to see the results of my dedication because it gave me a feeling of accomplishment.

July 31 [continued]: *On July 30, between 1:00 and 5:00 P.M. I started making appointments for a local entrepreneur. He is also paying me hourly. So far, I've worked the following hours: Tuesday (July 30), four hours; Wednesday (July 31), seven and a half hours. Thursday and Friday I plan to work full days.*

As I continued this journal entry, my writing got progressively larger and sloppier. I vividly remember not being able to write my thoughts down fast enough. If I didn't get them out of my mind, I thought I would burst. Having a release during these challenging episodes is vital. My journal served this purpose because I wanted to avoid driving my husband and friends away by talking and talking. A bipolar support group would have been a great supplement to my journal. But because bipolar disorder was not discussed in the early 1990s as it is today, I was not aware that support groups existed. Because I had managed my symptoms for over ten years while on medication, I assumed I could manage them without. During periods of mania and depression I was determined to cope with the symptoms, so I turned to my husband, doctors, family, and friends to help give me perspective. Today, I am a member of a peer-led support group.

My hypomanic phases while off medication were characterized by milder manic symptoms. The primary symptoms I experienced included a racing mind, pressure to talk, difficulty sleeping and concentrating, and an excessive drive to be productive. Although these symptoms were milder compared to those of a full-blown manic phase, they were uncomfortable and intense. My drive to be productive ignited additional hypomanic symptoms. I felt as if I were trapped in a vicious cycle.

July 31 [continued]: *Last night I was awake between 3:30 and 5:30 A.M. I had to get up at 7:00 this morning, so I couldn't catch up by sleeping later. I got up and read because I couldn't quit thinking. The night before, I had dreams that I was scheduling appointments all night long. These are both danger signs—warnings. I know I have to work full days tomorrow and Friday, but after that (we'll be on vacation August 3–10) I've got to pace myself.*

I dreaded sleeping at night when I was in a hypomanic phase. I felt as if I had no control over my turbulent mind.

The following is a vivid description of a typical hypomanic sleep experience: I lie in bed, and although my eyes are shut, they feel wide open. I'm conscious of them moving erratically, trying to catch up to my unconnected thoughts. My mind seems to be a separate entity that thinks and plans nonstop. It won't release me from my thoughts, even though, intellectually, I know I need to sleep. I feel trapped and imprisoned. Other times I lie there with my eyes open as frustration engulfs me. When I am fortunate enough to sleep, it's not a deep sleep. My mind rarely shuts down.

My sleep cycle is very close to the surface. Sometimes I'll wake up during the night and wonder if I'm thinking in my dreams or if I'm still awake. I often wake up from a dream that seems so real that I convince myself to finish it.

Lack of sleep in and of itself can cause manic or depressive episodes. See Chapter 10 for tips on getting a good night's sleep.

July 31 [continued]: *There's a strong correlation between working long hours and loss of sleep—racing mind—always feeling as though I have to be doing something productive. Example: I worked from 8:30 A.M. to 6:00 P.M. today (by the time I finished my paperwork). From 6:45 to 9:30 P.M. Fred and I were at our child prep class—it's now 10:30 P.M. and I still have not relaxed. Goal: Try not to be so driven—relax. Take time for me, especially before going to bed—it will help me sleep.*

A journal will help you to identify the areas you need to work on due to medication changes. Make it your goal to focus on the cause and effect of your behaviors and actions. Talk to your partner, family, doctors, and friends about solutions. Be open-minded about their suggestions.

Fred noted the following:

One of Kristin's challenges during pregnancy was to limit her working hours. I often had to tell her to stop working and unwind. Documenting her appointments, planning her day, and writing in her journal could wait until tomorrow. It was time to call it a day at nine o'clock at night!

Kristin listened and stopped working within ten to fifteen minutes, most of the time. Occasionally, after a half-hour, she was still writing furiously so I would then insist that she stop what she was doing.

Fred and I had a relaxing vacation from August 3 to 10 at my parents' "up north" vacation property on Lake Michigan. We spend time there as often as we can because it's beautiful and peaceful—it's our haven. The timing for this vacation was ideal because I needed a reprieve from my work. I didn't even feel the need to write in my journal while I was on vacation. That's an indication that I did not need to manage my thoughts. What a contrast from how I was feeling on July 31. Nothing could have kept me from communicating my racing and chaotic thoughts that night.

Going on vacation helped me to rearrange my outlook. It enabled me to concentrate on things other than work—like enjoying life. Imagine that!

Fred added the following observation:

> Our vacation the first week of August came at a good time. Kristin had been working too many hours and needed time away from her job. Summers are also busy and stressful for me in my profession, which made the timing perfect. We didn't think about work or keeping a schedule. We just enjoyed the sun and the beach, campfires, and other relaxing activities.

Find a place where you can go to get away from your everyday routine. If you cannot take a week off for a vacation getaway, consider taking a Friday or a Monday off to extend your weekend. If staying home works best, plan activities that you enjoy doing. Be creative. Scheduling quality time takes initiative and preparation. The benefits will be fulfilling and long lasting.

August 9: The last week of July, Roscoe's kicks were definitely stronger. I was in my twenty-second week. I like to lie down and feel the "Roscoe Ballet." On occasion (usually when I don't have much food in my stomach) I get really nauseous, dizzy, and hot. Drinking a protein drink helps me. Other than that, I feel pretty good.

This past week (week 23) I started to feel a lot of pressure in my stomach and pelvic floor [it's not really my stomach, but when I was pregnant, I often referred to my growing uterus as my stomach]. *My stomach has grown a lot during the past few weeks. I'm finally starting to look pregnant.*

This made me happy, because until that point, I thought I looked as if I was simply gaining weight due to overeating. It was a whole new adventure once people started noticing that I was pregnant.

August 12: I played golf August 5 and 9. On August 9, I hurt my back golfing and couldn't even finish the ninth hole. It was intense pain. It's been three days since then, and my back still hurts. Saturday I couldn't even bend over and pick anything up. It's still painful when I do everyday things. I canceled my golf league. I decided not to golf any more this season.

During our vacation, I spent time walking along Lake Michigan picking up Petoskey stones (Michigan's state stone). Looking for them was a fixation; focusing on their unique design among all the other stones was calming. I spent hours looking. However, bending over repeatedly to pick them up aggravated my back pain.

Moderation would have helped to prevent this. My back was susceptible to injury, and the twisting involved in golf exacerbated my pain. If you are doing anything during your pregnancy that's painful or irritating, stop doing it. Remember that your muscles are even more prone to injury while you're pregnant. Benefit from my mistakes.

Keep in mind that people who are bipolar have an increased tendency to live in the moment, without regard for future consequences. Because I didn't listen to the initial nagging pain in my back, it became a problem that had a negative effect during and after my pregnancy. My goal is to increase your awareness so that you can apply it to your own unique circumstances.

August 19: My back is still bothering me. Sitting at my desk working for over four hours a day makes the pain more intense. When I go out to eat [which is one of my favorite things to do because it involves eating and visiting], *sitting in one place aggravates my back pain to the point that it becomes my number one focus. I'm thankful Roscoe gives me a diversion. He is kicking more and more. I love to feel him kick and move around!*

August 31: My back continues to hurt. Last night it hurt a lot during the night. I couldn't sleep much. I needed a heating pad.

September 7: I have severe back pain (same spot) today. I spent five hours at a family reunion. Sitting straight up with no support [we ate and visited at picnic tables] *and standing really hurts. Fred and I walked for one hour and twenty minutes this evening. My right knee really hurts, especially when I sit or stand up.*

Moderation was definitely lacking here. Think about the areas in your life in which you might not show moderation in your behaviors or actions. Write them down in your pregnancy journal and share them with your partner, trusted friends, or doctors. Give them permission ahead of time to help you keep your life balanced during this unpredictable time. Do your best to accept their feedback and implement their suggestions.

September 11 (tomorrow I'll begin my twenty-ninth week): For the past couple of weeks I've felt a strong (knotted-up feeling) pressure in my uterus (my lower abdominal area). I thought it was Roscoe changing positions. A friend told me that I'm probably feeling Braxton Hicks contractions. My ob-gyn agreed. I feel a lot of pressure for about ten to fifteen seconds, although it doesn't hurt. They occur regularly.

Braxton Hicks contractions are intermittent painless uterine contractions. They can occur after the third month; they help to prepare the uterus for delivery. However, lower abdominal pressure and cramping can also be a sign of preterm labor. Check with your ob-gyn to be sure.

Write down any significant physical changes you notice in your pregnancy journal. If you need an explanation about the change, call your ob-gyn or ask at your next appointment for clarification. Keeping track of these changes will increase your involvement in your baby's development.

September 23: On September 16, my child prep instructor told me that Roscoe had the hiccups. [I couldn't figure out why my stomach was moving up and down regularly.] *He also had them on September 18. It's a weird feeling.*

September 30: Yesterday, for the first time, I felt Roscoe's specific body parts. I felt a hand or foot sticking out. It was an extraordinary feeling.

My back continues to hurt—persistently. On September 19, I saw an orthopedic surgeon about my back [a self-referral]. *He told me that I had sprained my dorsal/thoracic spine area and gave me a brochure that included back stretching and strengthening exercises. They take about forty-five minutes to do. I did them every other day (half in the morning and half in the evening) from September 19 to 30. The pain did not decrease at all. My shoulder blade area (trigger point) feels aggravated.*

A trigger point is an area that, when stimulated, will initiate an attack of neuralgia. Neuralgia is severe, sharp pain that occurs along the course of a nerve. It is caused by pressure on nerve trunks, faulty nerve nutrition, toxins, or inflammation. Prior knowledge of this definition would have provided me with true validation and understanding of this pain. I was fully aware of the intense, chronic pain I felt, yet I was uncertain about its true origin—I knew it was real but wasn't sure if it was exaggerated by my bipolar imagination.

During the months I was off lithium, I consistently questioned my judgment and perception. It's likely that you will also encounter challenges or obstacles during this period. Seek information to help you understand and overcome them. Knowledge will validate you, and that always feels great.

September 30 [continued]: *It feels as if knives are in my back, especially when I sit in a chair. The sprain seems to have traveled down the left part of my back. I continue to use a heating pad daily. At least two times a week, I have trouble sleeping because of the intense pain. Saturday and Sunday, September 28 and 29, we were again staying at my parents' vacation property, celebrating our wedding anniversary. We went to a nice restaurant Saturday, and the pain in my back was almost unbearable. I was in extreme pain all weekend.*

On October 2 I had an appointment with a doctor at a pain clinic. I initiated this appointment as well. Maybe it was a way of exerting control in what seemed like a hopeless situation. I was desperate to get relief from this constant pain. It interfered with my daily activities, increased my stress level, and affected me emotionally. Stress can ignite mania.

October 2: The doctor I saw diagnosed me as having myofascial pain in my left shoulder. He said that was causing the sprainlike feeling in my middle and lower left side as well. For example, my back hurts when I roll over in bed or when I check my blind spot while driving. He referred me to a physical therapist.

I was immediately encouraged because I knew that I could actively participate in the solution to the problem that was dominating my life. Going to physical therapy was another way for me to increase control over my life. As I mentioned earlier, for me, being off medication was the antithesis of control. For unique situations in your life, make a conscious effort to regain some control. It will give you a feeling of accomplishment and satisfaction.

October 7: I saw my physical therapist on October 2, 4, and 7. She starts each session (which usually lasts about forty-five minutes) with seven minutes of ultrasound that she applies to my "trigger area." [The ultrasound waves are converted to heat in the muscle. The heat increases circulation.] *She told me that on October 2, I had a muscle mass the size of a lemon under my left shoulder blade. No wonder my back hurts so much!* [I felt affirmed knowing that there was a physical reason for it.] *Today it was only the size of a large marble. She shows me new exercises during every visit. I do them twice a day. They take between fifteen and twenty minutes per session (A.M. and P.M.).* [I was diligent about doing my back exercises and stretches. I would have done anything to make the anguish go away.] *She ends each appointment by putting an ice pack on my back for twenty minutes. I've been icing my back three to four times a day since October 2.*

I'm noticing a big improvement already. October 4–6, I slept on my left side for the first time in weeks. The sprain feeling is lessening. I still feel as if I have knives under my shoulder blade, but the pain has decreased a lot. My back felt OK today, but it hurt during child prep class. It also hurt a little throughout the night.

October 14: My back is getting better.

My spirits were lifted as I experienced improvement. I started believing that my agony was almost over. It was helpful to look at previous journal entries to remind myself that this pain was temporary. I had lots of entries to review because keeping track of my progress helped me to cope with the pain and provided me with an outlet. (Many excerpts have been omitted here.) Try this strategy during your pregnancy. It can help you to manage and overcome any complications.

October 19: Fred and I went out with friends tonight. My trigger area didn't hurt, but my back started to feel sore after dinner. Sprainlike feeling.

October 21–23: My back is feeling much better. October 21, my therapist had me start using the arm machine [upper body ergometer—UBE] *for five minutes to strengthen my back. She wants me to start getting back to my normal routine. Example: Work at my desk for one hour at a time.*

She was specific so that I would not go overboard.

October 24: I am now at thirty-five weeks. I continue to go to physical therapy three times a week. My therapist uses ultrasound under my shoulder blade for seven minutes every visit. The mass is practically gone. She recommended that I continue doing my back stretches and strengthening exercises for fifteen minutes twice a day [even when I'm tempted to skip them]. *I make time to apply the ice pack three times a day. It's fantastic to see such improvement. I've been sleeping much better as well.*

Fred noted the following:

When Kristin first injured her back, she stopped exercising, lifting heavy objects, and simply rested it. We thought it would get better. However, when there was no improvement, I was relieved that she went to a physical therapist. Even though it was time-consuming and inconvenient, her back responded to the treatment. I knew that being eight months' pregnant made her feel uncomfortable, but she didn't need severe back pain as well.

October 24 [continued]: *I've been feeling pretty good lately. Roscoe's so active. We call him Roscoe "the piglet" because he seems to be taking up all the room in my stomach—from top to bottom, side to side. Today I went on a walk and started feeling lots of pressure in my lower abdomen. Roscoe's getting so big!*

Now that my back is healing, I continue to exercise about five times a week. I did aerobics the last two Tuesdays. I'll keep exercising until I deliver. I've gained twenty-five pounds. I'm so glad my back is getting better, so I can keep exercising regularly.

October 25: My back feels great today. I sat at my desk scheduling appointments. It was the first time in ages that I have not made calls from my recliner. From 5:00 to 9:00 P.M. I had dinner with a friend and then visited with other friends. I had no problem with my back. At 4:00 P.M. I had gone to physical therapy. I'm up to ten minutes on the arm machine.

October 26: Fred and I drove to visit friends who live near Chicago. It took about four hours to get there. Saturday evening we went to the October Festival. I had excruciating back pain. We got back to their house around 10:30 P.M.

During my pregnancy, I continued to keep in contact with my friends—some knew about my bipolar disorder, and others did not. Looking back, I'm glad I did not hibernate at home. Fred and I attempted to live our lives to the fullest.

If you decide to try to have a baby, your life doesn't necessarily have to be on hold for many months. However, you might have to adapt and make adjustments to your individual needs. Look at it as a temporary challenge with a wonderful reward.

October 29: I still use the arm machine at physical therapy for ten minutes. I've increased my back exercises, using an elastic band (Thera-Band), to eighteen repetitions each. My back is getting stronger.

October 30: Appointment with Dr. Hiemenga. Summary: Roscoe is lying sideways across my stomach [transverse]. *If he's still sideways next week, I'll need an ultrasound. If the ultrasound confirms that he's sideways, they'll have to try to move him while he's inside my stomach* [this is called an "external version"]. *Next week, during my thirty-seventh week, I'll go to the hospital's labor and delivery unit. They will give me Brethine, a medication (she told me it would make me feel jittery), and then try to move the baby. There is a small chance I'll go into premature labor.* [My due date is November 28—Thanksgiving Day. The doctor told me to bring my overnight bag just in case.] *If I do go into premature labor, Dr. Hiemenga will deliver our baby. Everything else looks great!*

November 1: I started feeling Braxton Hicks contractions at 3:45 P.M. Since they became regular and lasted so long, at 9:15 P.M. the doctor on call told me to go to Labor and Delivery. We found out that Roscoe's now breech (buttocks down), still not a good position for delivery. I have to take Brethine every six hours to stop contractions until my next appointment, Wednesday, November 6. The doctor told me I have to take it easy until then—no exercise or walks.

November 10: What a tough week—especially Tuesday. My temperature was over 100. The Brethine gave me side effects—headache, nausea, and a racing heartbeat. I've had trouble breathing, I can't catch my breath, and I cough a lot. Sleeping (or lying down to rest) makes it worse. Tomorrow is the external version. Roscoe moves all the time, and I'll miss that after he's born!

In *What to Expect When You're Expecting,* Murkoff, Eisenberg, and Hathaway (2002) describe an external version this way:

The most frequently used and medically conventional approach to turning a fetus to a head-down position is external cephalic version (ECV), in which a physician attempts, with ultrasound guidance, to gently shift the fetus by applying his or her hands to the mother's abdomen. The condition of the fetus must be monitored continuously to be sure the umbilical cord isn't accidentally compressed or the placenta disturbed. The procedure is best performed in the hospital before labor begins or very early in labor, when the uterus is still relatively relaxed.

The more relaxed the uterus is, in fact, the more likely ECV is to be successful (which is why ECV works better in second and subsequent pregnancies than in first). Researchers are looking into the possibility that giving an epidural to women undergoing ECV may also increase the chances that the procedure will successfully turn their babies. Once turned, most fetuses stay head down, but a few do revert to breech before delivery. When successful (as it is more than half the time), ECV can reduce the likelihood that a cesarean delivery will be necessary. (page 293)

November 11: My external version was a success today. What a blessing. I was first given IV Brethine. It made me feel as if I had had ten cups of coffee. Dr. Hiemenga described the procedure by telling me to imagine pulling my upper lip over my head. She and a resident moved Roscoe simultaneously. It only took about a minute, but it was immensely painful.

Fred told me that I squeezed his hand like a vise. Here's what he had to say about the process:

When I went with Kristin for the external version, I didn't know what to expect. I had no idea how they were going to turn our baby. Was Kristin going to be sedated or put under anesthesia? How many people would be involved in the procedure? When I found out what would take place, I knew all I could do was hold Kristin's hand, try to keep her calm, and offer moral support. I knew the procedure was painful for her, but thankfully it only lasted a short time and was successful on the first try. I was relieved when it worked, and I hoped that Roscoe wouldn't turn upside down again before the birth took place.

My ECV is an example of a procedure that might be necessary during a pregnancy. It's possible that you will experience other medical difficulties. It's important for you to gather all the information you can for any procedure that is recommended. Only then can you and your partner make an informed decision on what is best for you. Remember to always ask for help and support if and when you need it.

SUMMARY

The following steps will help you to manage and cope with your pregnancy and the subsequent birth of your baby:

- Purchase a book on pregnancy, such as *What to Expect When You're Expecting,* to use as a reference guide.

- Adjust your work or personal schedule to decrease stress.

- Continue to exercise—in moderation—to keep healthy and to manage your possible mania or depression. Physical therapy facilities are sometimes good sources for prenatal exercise classes.

- Contact your area hospitals/birthing centers about different birthing options.

- Talk with your psychiatrist, psychologist, social worker, or counselor to help you monitor and process your bipolar symptoms.

- After consulting with your doctors, consider resuming medication, if necessary.

- Continue to write in your pregnancy journal to manage and cope with bipolar symptoms.

- Record information about each prenatal appointment to help monitor your pregnancy.

- During difficult times, seek help and guidance.

- Trust others to help you.

- Tell your doctors if you're not getting enough sleep.

- Maintain connections with friends and family.

- Become part of the solution to your challenges.

- Maintain organization and structure.

- Strive to maintain a balanced life.

- Set realistic goals.

- Continue to reduce stress—stress ignites mania.

- Remain focused during your labor and delivery. A labor coach is essential.

Chapter 6

Nearing the Finish Line

With each passing day we grew more eager to meet our new baby. The following two journal entries relate the indications that our baby would soon be born.

November 16: When I was at the movie theater today, it felt as if Roscoe dropped. I felt lots of pressure on my pelvic floor.

November 26: Today at my doctor's appointment I found out that Roscoe's head is engaged. [Roscoe's head is in the proper position, ready for birth.]

My due date was in two days. I was like a marathon runner who sees the last mile marker. I could visualize holding our baby in my arms.

Once you are pregnant, there is a finite number of days (approximately 280) until the birth of your baby. For those of you who struggle with bipolar symptoms due to medication changes, seek comfort in knowing that it's temporary. You will treasure your baby and the love that he or she brings forever.

Picture yourself at the end of the pregnancy. You might encounter challenges for which you're not prepared. That's common in any pregnancy. I've done my best to provide you with coping skills to help manage them. My biggest challenge, in addition to managing my bipolar symptoms, was chronic back pain. I want to emphasize the importance of seeking help and finding a solution to any challenge that arises during your pregnancy.

During these nine months, focus on the relationships with your loved ones. Make the most of your current family situation. Once a parent, you're always a parent. On my grandpa's ninetieth birthday, he took his "kids" out to dinner (ages sixty-four, sixty-two, and fifty-six). Your kids will always be your kids; however, they do grow up and move away. Once they're living on their own, you'll still have your friends and other loved ones. Keep those relationships alive and well.

Throughout your pregnancy, continue to mentally prepare for life with your new baby. There will be significant changes in your daily routine once the baby is born. Although having structure is beneficial for bipolars, learning to be flexible is crucial.

Because so much of my energy was focused on managing my bipolar symptoms during pregnancy, I didn't get overly stressed out about "the small stuff." For example: How do I know these are real labor pains? Will I get to the hospital on time? Will I be able to fit into the clothes I want to wear home? Will we have too much company? Will my mother take over—she's spending the first *week* with us? After all, I am the mom. You get the idea.

Making it to the end of the pregnancy was my main focus. I knew that we could handle the delivery process. I was also confident that we could care for our newborn.

During the course of the pregnancy, preparing for Roscoe's arrival was a milestone we had been dying to reach. Buying clothes and necessities for him brightened our days. I have a confession to make that I'm embarrassed to admit. Although my ultimate goal was to have a safe pregnancy and a healthy baby, and I would have been elated to give birth to either a boy or a girl, I secretly wanted to have a girl. Because of this feeling, I convinced myself that I was going to have a boy. We decorated Roscoe's room with unisex colors and bought him unisex clothes, including an adorable blue and red Mickey Mouse snowsuit. I didn't allow myself to buy our baby anything pink.

Just for fun, Fred took a picture of me prior to Roscoe's birth, holding Pampers diapers (made for boys) that I had purchased. I knew that if we had a boy, Fred and I would be filled with joy. If our baby was a girl, my secret wish would have come true. It was a win-win situation for me. I wanted to protect myself from feeling anything but complete happiness when we found out the sex of our baby. Referring to our unborn baby as Roscoe also prepared me for giving birth to a boy.

December 1: Fred and I are eagerly waiting for Roscoe. It feels as if he's dropped even lower. When I sit down it feels as if I'm supporting a shelf (my lower abdomen). We're getting anxious—we want to meet our baby!

December 6: Fred and I are more than ready for baby Roscoe's grand appearance. I'm past the point of waking up each day wondering, is Roscoe coming today? It's much easier for me to take one day at a time, realizing that he has to come sooner or later. I continue to feel great.

Last week I started getting a little uptight about a couple of things [the delivery and upcoming changes in our lives. Here's what I did about it]. *Sunday, December 1, was the turning point in terms of my attitude. I went through my* Portals of Prayer [daily devotions] *books from 1987 to the present (the ones that I kept) and tore out each one that had special significance to me. Many of them focused on giving your worries to God, comfort, and prayer. I've been reading a few of them daily, along with the suggested Bible verse. Now that I'm reminded that God's in control of everything (concerning Roscoe's arrival), I feel a sense of peace. Fred and I are looking forward to seeing Roscoe. I love Roscoe so much—already! I have been feeling terrific! I'm uncomfortable, but other than that, I've been doing well.*

Fred made the following comments:

Kristin and I were trying to be patient waiting for our baby to be born. At that point, he was over a week late and I guess he was just being stubborn. I knew Kristin was uncomfortable physically. I remember her telling me she felt as if she had a twenty-five-pound bag of dog food tied to the front of her. Her mental attitude was great. She had been reading passages from *Portals of Prayer* and I could see the difference in her. She put things in God's hands and didn't worry about all the details that were part of having her first baby.

During pregnancy, there will be times that you will feel worried and overwhelmed—that's normal. People who have bipolar disorder (and even those who don't) often fixate on their worries. It's important not to let them triumph over you. Fight back! I did, and you can too—with the help of your pregnancy journal. It can help you to manage anxiety.

The first step in defeating your worries is to identify them and write them in your journal. It will help you to figure out an action plan instead of obsessing about them. You'll find that some of your concerns even seem silly once you see them on paper. Talking with your supporters can also provide you with ways to conquer fears. Try to surround yourself with positive, encouraging people. Go ahead and take charge; putting worries into perspective feels wonderful.

It's interesting that a person's perception often dominates his or her reality. Fill your mind with optimistic thoughts. Go to the bookstore or library and get a book that focuses on positive thinking. Changing my perspective was the most important thing I did to change my attitude. I figured this out on my own, and it made a significant difference in the outcome of the days leading up to Roscoe's birth. I felt peace rather than anxiety.

December 4: I have been extremely productive during the past few days. I'm sure it's due to the nesting instinct that I've heard and read about.

The surge of energy was incredible. Knowing that our baby's birth was imminent, I realized I had one last chance to prepare.

I completed my work, bought additional necessities for Roscoe, and cleaned the house.

The journal entries below, dated December 7 and 8, were written soon after the birth of our baby. I felt compelled to update the labor and delivery aspects of this journey.

The evening of December 7, nine days past my due date, I called my mom to chat. During our conversation I unknowingly described having ruptured membranes. I started showing signs of this on December 4, but I didn't mention it to Fred. Even though I had read *What to Expect When You're Expecting,* I still thought my water would break all at once or that it would be obvious. I had envisioned it happening in public. It didn't occur to me that a slow trickle counted; I figured this was just part of the pregnancy experience. Logic had escaped me. My mom told me to immediately call Dr. Hiemenga. She emphasized that once the membranes rupture, there is an increased chance of infection for me and the baby.

Always mention even seemingly minor things to your doctor or medical professional during your pregnancy. Let him or her determine the significance of your concern. I was fortunate to have a mom who is knowledgeable about pregnancy. Her professional background was a bonus. Search for a similar person. It's helpful to get feedback from experienced people.

December 7: I was admitted to the hospital at 11:00 P.M. Amniotic fluid has been leaking since December 4. The nurse who monitored my contractions said they were pretty strong. I slept in a birthing bed and only got about three hours of sleep. I woke up at 7:00 A.M.

I was nervous but mentally prepared to start the labor process as soon as I arrived the evening of December 7. To add to my apprehension, they told me I had to wait until 7:00 A.M. before they would induce labor with oxytocin (Pitocin). I remember feeling disappointed because I wanted to start labor immediately to avoid worrying about the effects of Pitocin. I had heard that it can intensify contractions. Dr. Hiemenga said Pitocin can be used to start labor and intensify contractions, making them stronger, longer, and potentially more regular.

December 8: The Pitocin drip started at 8:30 A.M. My contractions came hard and fast. I wanted pain medication by noon, but waited until 2:00 P.M. The Phenergen and Statol that I was given to reduce my pain didn't help at all. At that point, I was dilated to only 2 centimeters.

I recall wondering how I could feel consistent, long, excruciating contractions and only be dilated to 2 centimeters. I reread the *Portals of Prayer* devotions that I had brought with me until I could not understand the words because of the intense pain. I was certain I looked silly to the nurses and residents, reading them between contractions, but I didn't care. They gave me strength.

Staying focused and doing breathing exercises helped me to get through my contractions. *Hee, hee, hoo* was my favorite, even though it sounded ridiculous to me when we learned it in our child prep class. I also listened to music that I brought from home and focused on a football game that Fred was casually watching. This was proof that I needed a distraction, something to focus on, because my eyes were glued to every play. The last time I watched football had been the Super Bowl, nearly a year ago!

Fred was an exceptional coach during my labor and delivery. He was receptive to my needs and supported me throughout the entire process. Sometimes his silent presence was most helpful—especially when I was concentrating on my breathing exercises during contractions. For some reason, I didn't like it when he tried to help me count during contractions. I remember saying, "Don't help me count!" Talk with your labor coach ahead of time about your expectations. You'll tell them your specific needs as you labor, sometimes minute by minute.

December 8 [continued]: *I was at my pain threshold by 3:00 P.M. Dr. Burke* [the doctor on call] *recommended an epidural. Relief at last! My contractions felt like strong menstrual cramps instead of the excruciating contractions that had previously been coming so fast and hard. I started pushing at 9:30 P.M. and continued to push until 11:53 P.M.*

My mom arrived at 10:30 P.M. I told her that she could come into the birthing room, but I emphasized my need to continue concentrating. I was so focused that I couldn't stop and visit with her, but she understood. It was comforting to see her sitting across the room.

During labor and delivery, do what's best for you. Don't worry about the wants and needs of others. Your goal is to do the best you can to bring your baby into the world.

I was told to push three times per contraction. I didn't have the opportunity to rest between contractions, which were three minutes apart. Because I was so determined and focused, I pushed four times during every contraction. I quickly understood why people refer to it as labor. I cannot emphasize enough how important it is to have a labor support person, such as your partner, family member, or a friend. The encouragement is priceless.

Fred described the process as follows:

> Kristin's labor seemed like an eternity. I got to the hospital at 8:00 A.M. as they were getting ready to start Pitocin. The pain was unbearable for her around noon, and finally at 3:00 P.M. she got her epidural. This helped her relax some, but the contractions were still painful. The last two and a half hours were the most intense. I tried my best to keep Kristin as comfortable as possible. I put cool compresses on her forehead because pushing a big baby out is hard work.

Beautiful Katherine was finally born. What a blessing! When Dr. Burke told us that we had a girl, I was completely shocked. I said, "I can't believe it's a girl!" Holding Katherine for the first time was incredible. Immediately she looked into my eyes, and I felt a surge of joy. Fred eventually went home, and my mom spent the night in my room with me. We went to sleep at 4:30–5:00 A.M.

Fred recalls how he felt that night:

> When Katherine was finally born late in the evening on December 8, there was pure joy in my heart. Taking part in her birth was one of the most memorable experiences in my life. Holding her for the first time was just terrific!
>
> I have been a runner for a long time and have run six marathons.

After Katherine was finally born, I told Kristin what she went through made a marathon look like a walk in the park.

Thinking back to the first meeting we had at the genetics clinic, I realize that the decisions we made, the risks we took, and working our way through this pregnancy were enormous challenges. Katherine's arrival made them all worthwhile!

This pregnancy experience brought on a kaleidoscope of emotions: apprehension, trust, joy, anxiety, pain, love, peace, and laughter. It helped prepare me for my second pregnancy, which was much easier.

The last section of this chapter was written by my mother, Marjorie McCulloch, who is a registered nurse.

A Mother's Observations

We were so excited! Any day we'd be grandparents. I was determined not to forget that this was the beginning of Kristin and Fred's new life. We got the news that they were admitted to the hospital and that labor would be induced the next morning. We stayed close to the phone. At about 7:00 P.M. the call came, saying that labor was progressing slowly and that Katherine would no doubt arrive before midnight. My bag was packed and I was ready for the two-hour drive to the hospital. David (Kristin's dad) planned to join us the next day. I got to the labor and delivery unit at 10:30 P.M.

I hadn't planned to be in the delivery room, so I asked the

receptionist if I could go to the door and let them know I'd be in the waiting room. When Kristin heard my voice, she said I could come in. I was thrilled! I'd loved working labor and delivery as a nurse—it's where I was working part time when Kristin was born.

I spent the next hour and a half as a quiet observer, sometimes sitting in an easy chair out of the way or taking a peek from the end of the delivery table. I could not have been more impressed with Kristin and Fred and how they were working together. The doctor and the labor and delivery staff were also on the team. With each push, Katherine's head would come down the birth canal, only to slip back up between contractions. Little did we know that there would be much more laboring before she made her grand entrance.

At one point, the nurse quietly asked me, "How can you be so calm? Most mothers would be a basket case watching their daughter labor like this." I was praying hard, knowing that all the team players were competent and that things were under control.

Katherine finally arrived, and in my opinion she couldn't have been more beautiful. She weighed 9 pounds, 13 ounces and was 20 inches long. Fred, who was worn out, went home for a quiet night's sleep. I stayed with Kristin, who was both ecstatic and exhausted. She had remained focused and determined until Katherine was born.

The next morning when we were talking, we figured out that Katherine had been born after 300 pushes. Here's how we came up with that number:

- Kristin pushed for two and a half hours.

- Contractions every two minutes equals thirty per hour.

- She pushed four times per contraction rather than the three that the doctor and nurse had recommended. The extra push was because she had the energy and wanted to meet her new baby as soon as possible. Four pushes times thirty contractions per hour thus equals 120 pushes per hour.

- Finally, 120 pushes per hour for two and a half hours equals 300 pushes.

I'd forgotten that all this was written down in typical "Kristin" fashion. I came across her notes recently as I was going through the things I'd saved after Katherine's birth.

Chapter 7

Déjà Vu:
My Second Pregnancy

M anaging my second pregnancy was also challenging, but I had the advantage of a successful first experience to guide me. I kept track of my cycles regularly, so I knew when I was ovulating. I also understood the importance of getting pregnant as soon as possible once I was lithium free.

Katherine was almost two when we decided to have another baby. Taking care of a toddler was thus an added responsibility that we did not have the first time. Having Katherine in our life reminded us of what we were striving for—another daughter or a son. I was fortunate, once again, to get pregnant right away.

I wrote the following summary in my journal.

April 3, 1994: January 27, I woke up at 4:30 A.M. with a wave of nausea. It lasted for one to two hours. My period is due January 28. Fred and I did a pregnancy test January 30; it was faintly positive. We did a second pregnancy test February 2, and the positive line was much darker.

We were excited to reach this first milestone. My new focus was managing this pregnancy along with the added responsibility of caring for a two-year-old.

I continued doing aerobics, lifting weights, and walking regularly throughout my pregnancy and kept a record of each workout. It gave me a feeling of accomplishment and a positive boost of energy. My addiction to exercise trumped my judgment, however, and I began to exercise excessively. Moderation was difficult for me.

April 3 [continued]: *Soon after I got pregnant, I strained my back while exercising and began physical therapy on February 17. My primary* [physical] *therapist has a lot of experience working with pregnant women. I started out going three times per week, and now I only go once a month.*

I'm still nauseous from morning until night. I hate this feeling! It's not as bad as it was with Katherine, but I feel imprisoned by it. I can't wait until I feel better [I knew that I would].

I managed this pregnancy differently from the way I managed my first one. My life was much busier with a toddler. Occasionally, I would write in my pregnancy journal, but I relied mostly on my calendar to keep my life organized. I didn't go anywhere without it. I always made sure that each day was planned before I went to sleep, because organization and structure were important to me during this unpredictable time.

Katherine went to day care three days a week, which she enjoyed, while I sold advertising part time for a business directory.

Katherine occasionally modeled for an agency, so that kept me busy juggling our schedule to accommodate last-minute auditions and jobs. Handling stress was an ongoing challenge.

On February 10, I started a yoga class to help me reduce stress and learn relaxation techniques. I had to quit after two sessions because I was too nauseous to participate in many of the exercises. Eating saltine crackers in class to help decrease my nausea was awkward and ineffective. The hardest part of the class was trying to relax my mind and body. Attempting to quiet the thoughts in my head was torture. The instructor encouraged us to relax each body part, including our minds. For me that was like trying to silence the noise at a NASCAR race.

In March, I had an insatiable desire to find out more about my bipolar disorder. Prior to the onset of my behavioral changes at age thirteen, I was well balanced, conscientious, trustworthy, and conservative. I was eager to please my parents and teachers and became upset if anyone even looked at me with disapproval.

Questions about my past came at me faster than I could process them. When did I transform into the girl I was ashamed of for so many years? Did something happen years ago that precipitated this condition? Was I manic first, or depressed? I knew that I experienced periods of both mania and depression, but I had no idea how long each lasted; was it days, weeks, or months? Did a particular event trigger the drastic change in me from mania to depression, or were the transformations random? I set everything else aside when Katherine was at day care to find the answers to these questions, which held my mind hostage.

I knew that the answers could be found in the diaries I kept from ages ten to twenty. I read and studied both of the five-year diaries that I completed from January 1, 1973, to December 31, 1982. This ten-year period covers the following stages and personal experiences in my life:

- Childhood

- The onset of bipolar disorder

- Coping methods prior to treatment

- Descriptive experiences of mania and depression

- Subtle and obvious cries for help

- Medical and psychological treatment attempts and my willingness to get better

- Desperate attempts to manage my bipolar disorder on my own, months before I was diagnosed

- Diagnosis and treatment

- Coping with my new life

- Preparing for college

- Starting college in September 1980

- Adapting to college life while managing bipolar disorder

I read every page in both diaries for the first time since I had written them. I was determined to discover what had happened. I took a yellow pad of paper and copied every entry that I thought might hold a clue for me. Reading about my previous life was cathartic, uncomfortable, and scary—I felt as if the world had stopped; nothing was more important than understanding my past.

I'm not sure how many days it took to complete this mission, but I do know that I didn't stop until I was done. Discovering answers evoked many emotions: intrigue, guilt, resentment, understanding, and sadness. I felt bad for the girl (me) who was forced to endure a life beyond her control. I became hypomanic and revved up after reopening these old wounds.

Providing myself with windows of serenity helped me to get through this turbulent time. When Katherine was two, I started attending a women's group at my church called Challenges. We met every Wednesday morning from 9:30 to 11:00 to share experiences on raising children and on life in general. I looked forward to going each week because it gave me a sense of belonging.

As much as I liked the group, however, I didn't feel comfortable sharing my bipolar condition in this setting. Katherine was in day care on Wednesdays, and I felt guilty taking time away from my job, but I realized that it was important to have balance. I needed to do this for my peace of mind. I made it a priority to maintain my relationships with friends and relatives during this unstable time.

Maintaining connections with people you are close to is critical. On the days I didn't work, Katherine and I kept busy visiting friends and relatives, including my grandparents, who lived an hour away. We drove to see them once a month. I believe that spending time with Grandma and Grandpa and watching them interact with their great-granddaughter gave me periods of sheer peace.

Katherine and I also regularly visited an elderly friend who lived in a nursing home. The smile on her face when we entered her room was priceless. Keeping Katherine away from her knick-knacks was a never-ending task, but it was worth it. I lost myself during these visits, and it felt satisfying.

I would also have coffee with friends who had small children. The kids would play together while we talked. On the days that I worked, I often made time to have lunch with my girlfriends. I continued to ask my friends how I was doing without lithium. It was one of the few opportunities I had to talk about how I was *really* feeling. I had become so good at concealing my racing thoughts that my friends usually told me there wasn't much difference in my behavior. Sometimes that was frustrating for me; I couldn't believe that they were unaware of the battles I had to fight to appear to be "normal."

Finding a balance between doing what was in my best interest and what had to be accomplished seemed like an unattainable goal. Before I went off medication, Fred and I decided that I would begin a new career as an investment advisor representative. Although it was important for me to set goals and work toward them, learning a new business added to my stress level. You're probably thinking, "No kidding." Keeping track of dates and appointments during this busy time was therapeutic. It helped me to organize my life and keep on task.

On March 28 I began to study for the Michigan life and

health insurance exam. This is not an easy test to pass, even under ideal conditions. Getting a life insurance license was a pre-requisite for my career as an investment advisor. I wanted to familiarize myself with the information prior to attending the class in Grand Rapids, April 11–15. Learning new information was challenging for me while I was off lithium, and I was uncertain about my ability to concentrate and retain the material.

On April 11, from 8:30 A.M. to 5:00 P.M., I attended my first day of class. I was thankful that the nausea was subsiding. During class I took copious notes to help reinforce the concepts. By the end of class on the next day, I was feeling overwhelmed with the amount of material the instructor presented. After discussing this with her, I decided to concentrate on getting my life insurance license, so I withdrew from the health insurance portion of the class. I knew it was in my best interest to take that class another time. It felt good to make this decision on my own. My judgment was still intact. That's saying a lot for a bipolar off medication.

The next day the instructor was planning on focusing on health insurance, so I stayed home and studied. On April 14, I had class all day, and on April 15 the life insurance segment was from 1:00 to 3:00 P.M. It concluded with a practice exam.

Fred made the following observations:

I knew Kristin was excited about becoming an investment advi-sor and having her own business. However, I was concerned about how much work she would have to do to get her licenses. She told me about all the different concepts, formulas, and legal terms she had to know. I was glad she made the decision to temporarily pass on the health insurance portion of the exam. It reduced the amount of time she needed to study for her test and also decreased her overall stress level, which was high.

I was also happy she asked her doctor about her inability to sleep. Most of the time, while off medication, Kristin did a good job seeking help when she needed it.

April 15: I talked to Dr. Eerdmans and told her I was extremely stressed out because of this insurance class. She told me that bipolar disorder can affect concentration. She suggested a low dose of lithium (I'm in my second trimester). She mentioned that the earlier studies that link heart defects to lithium aren't necessarily valid. We had a good conversation. It was reassuring to talk with someone who could understand how hard it is for me to deal with stress. It seems to take over every aspect of my life.

At that time, I would not consider going on a low dose of lithium. I made the decision to live with the stress and tried to reduce it on my own. Fred agreed that this was best for me as well.

The decision to avoid medication during pregnancy might not be best for everyone. Because of the internal challenges I experienced while off lithium, I wonder, in retrospect, if it was the best decision for me. However, if Dr. Eerdmans had strongly believed that I needed to begin a low dose of lithium, I would have agreed, because I trusted her.

This is a good example of the importance of seeking the opinions of doctors and others who are helping you to manage and monitor yourself while you're off medication. It's essential to let them help you with your judgment. In other words, allow them to act as your prefrontal lobe, thus giving you the capacity to discern the true nature of a situation.

Studying excessively for my life insurance exam was one way that I tried to gain control. I studied the material covered in class, reviewed my notes, took practice tests, and wrote out the material that was difficult for me to conceptualize. I was determined to pass the test the first time. On April 22, I took the life insurance exam and missed a passing grade by one point. I felt disappointed, frustrated, and even cried (once I got in my car, of course). I promptly arranged to retake the exam on April 28. I was like a bulldozer; nothing could stop me from tackling this material again. Studying became my priority in addition to caring for Katherine, and, as a result, sleeping was nearly impossible.

During the night, my mind insisted on making every minute count—I could not escape from the material I had been absorbing. As I tried to sleep, I visualized facts and figures and answered test questions all night long. I talked to Dr. Hiemenga about this at a routine appointment, and she immediately prescribed 500 milligrams of Chloral Hydrate (a sleeping pill). I took it April 26–29 and was amazed and thankful that it shut my mind off so I could sleep.

I passed the life insurance exam on April 28 and was exhilarated and relieved. I was happy to focus on my family and pregnancy again.

If you have difficulty sleeping at night, talk with your doctor. The *NAMI Advocate* (Spring/Summer 2004) reported that a 2004 study by Yonkers et al. found that:

> Difficulty sleeping and anxiety are powerful triggers for the recurrence of episodes in bipolar disorder. Tranquilizers and sedatives, which help to regulate sleep, may reduce the risk of episodes during or after pregnancy. Medications that stay in the body the least amount of time are preferred. Sedatives and hypnotics are excreted in breast milk, but there have been few reports of complications due to their use. (p. 2)

I recorded all pertinent information at each prenatal visit during this pregnancy. I liked to compare the measurements and other facts with the ones I had recorded during my pregnancy with Katherine. Every time I had a prenatal appointment, I came prepared with a list of concerns or questions to ask Dr. Hiemenga or the doctor I saw at that particular appointment. I understood that my time there was limited and that I had to make every minute count.

I made a conscious effort to be succinct so I would stay on track and maintain a cohesive train of thought. Sometimes I would visualize myself being organized and competent, even on the days I was in disarray. It took immense concentration to filter my racing thoughts during these appointments. After all, here I was with an opportunity to talk with someone about how I was feeling; better yet, I was even asked to describe how I was feeling.

Dr. Hiemenga made me feel proud, accepted, and self-confident when she told me consistently, at various appointments, how well I was doing off lithium. It validated me.

Your relationships with your ob-gyn and psychiatrist are a crucial part of your pregnancy. As a bipolar, you have a unique situation, and I can't stress enough how important it is for you to feel comfortable and confident with your doctors. Working with professionals who are empathetic is wonderful. Keep looking until you find the right match for you.

In mid-May, I had an ultrasound. Fred, Katherine, and I were thrilled to see our baby. (We made a conscious effort to make Katherine an integral part of this pregnancy, to help prepare her for the significant lifestyle change that was coming.) It was exciting to see the baby move around.

Again, we didn't want to know our baby's sex. During this pregnancy, I knew that I would be equally happy with a boy or a girl. Fred and I agreed that we wanted to be surprised. Katherine was excited that she would soon be a big sister. Sharing this time together was important, especially because the next day I had to go out of town on business.

On Wednesday, May 18, I made the two-hour drive to Detroit for my preliminary 403(b) tax-sheltered annuity training. I was fortunate to have my dad spend one-to-one time instructing me. We also focused on the Michigan state retirement system so that I could assist educators with their pension options and other pertinent financial issues. The material was new to me and required a lot of concentration.

I spent two nights with my parents. I appreciated staying with them because I enjoyed their company and felt secure in my former home. I returned home after my training on May 20.

This hectic schedule eventually caught up with me. I found a peculiar but effective outlet for managing the racing thoughts that I desperately wanted to stop. Brace yourself—this might sound crazy! At that time, we had three completed videotapes of Katherine. I took each videotape and wrote down a summary of every event we had taped. Our VCR had a counter, so I was able to write down the numbers as a reference point to document the date and event that occurred on that part of the tape. I was extremely precise. Intellectually, I thought this would be an efficient way to know what was on each tape and how to quickly fast-forward to a specific section or date. It never occurred to me that our next VCR might not have a counter. I was living in the moment.

I'm not sure if I realized that doing this tedious task was a lifeline for my mental health. It gave me a feeling of accomplishment, reminded me of happy times, and provided me with a way to channel excessive thoughts. So do whatever calms you down and makes you feel good!

On July 5–8 (Tuesday through Friday) and July 12–15 (Tuesday through Friday), there was tax-sheltered annuity training in the Detroit area, so once again I stayed with my parents. By the end of the second week, I had filled up two notepads with new information. Taking detailed notes during class helped to calm my mind; it gave me a focus and an escape. Writing has always helped me to reduce stress.

As you can see, my life was not put on hold during my second pregnancy. Functioning without lithium was difficult but manageable. I was fortunate to function as well as I did. Preparing for my new career was a diversion and gave me a feeling of accomplishment. The flexibility in my schedule was a bonus.

It's important for you to have a backup plan if working becomes too stressful. You might want to consider working fewer hours, or maybe you won't be able to work at all. Explore your options ahead of time.

July 11: I had an appointment with Dr. Hiemenga. Katherine was exposed to chicken pox on June 30. Dr. Hiemenga told me I shouldn't be around Katherine for the rest of the week.

This happened on a Monday. Since neither Katherine nor I had been exposed to chicken pox before, Dr. Hiemenga explained the complications if I were to contract it. She gave me a blood test to determine if I was immune to chicken pox and told me that she would phone by the end of the week with the results. The timing was perfect, because on Tuesday I had to drive to the Detroit area to complete my initial training.

July 14: At 4:00 P.M. Dr. Hiemenga's nurse called and told me that the blood test results for my chicken pox immunities came back. I'm immune to it!

From July 30 through August 7, we went on vacation, which gave me the chance to relax and recharge my batteries.

August 9 was the first day of appointments in my new career. I scheduled a 9:30 A.M., an 11:30 A.M., and a 2:00 P.M. My dad and I had a productive day, and my self-confidence was heightened. He drove to my home often and worked with me until I became comfortable going on appointments by myself. He was a terrific mentor.

Appointment setting and follow-up were, and continue to be, pivotal to this business. My calendar was full of work and personal duties; it helped me to keep my life organized. I am the ultimate list maker; once I write something down, it frees my mind up so I don't have to keep track of details.

Toward the end of August, my back started to bother me, so on August 30 I began physical therapy about twice a week. I had back spasms September 15–29. They came without warning and left me in excruciating pain.

The previous May, I had scheduled an appointment with an exercise specialist whose background was in exercise physiology. She helped me to put together a weight-lifting program using the weight machines at my health club (I brought my previous exercise log for her to use as a guide). I took precautions during this pregnancy because I wanted to make sure that I was using each machine correctly. I avoided exercises that would aggravate my previous back injury.

September 20: Today was the last time I did my complete weight routine because it aggravated my back. I still lift weights with my 5-pound dumbbells and do stomach crunches three times a week. On September 14 our baby moved to a head-

down (floating) position. By September 19 our baby's head was engaged.

My due date was October 8. It was time to start focusing on preparing for our new baby.

September 29: Over the course of this pregnancy, I've felt pretty good. My ambition and drive pushed me into stressful working habits. Today I just finished organizing my files and office. Dad and I had our last three appointments on September 27. I still have to follow up with a few prospective clients within the next week or so.

My goal was to stop working after Labor Day, but Dad and I are on a roll, and I don't want to break this rhythm. We have secured business with the majority of the people we've seen. Dad has been great to work with—he has good follow-up [skills], too. I couldn't feel better about changing careers. This job is challenging, but I know I'll succeed.

The only time my mind races and I notice manic behavior is when Dad and I have appointments. It takes a lot of time and energy to prepare for each one. Following up with clients requires organization and dedication. It can be all-consuming. I'm looking forward to going back on lithium.

On September 27, Dad and I had three appointments—a 3:15, a 5:00, and a 6:30. I had constant Braxton Hicks contractions from 4:15 to 9:00 P.M. If it had been my first pregnancy, I would have gone into the hospital for false labor. It seemed that everything was going in fast motion—as if I were in a human pressure cooker. Now that I've forced myself to stop working, I'm doing much better.

It's time to take a break from my job, and I've been working hard to make sure everything turns out perfectly. I want it all to be in place before the baby arrives.

To keep me busy when I'm not working (prior to having our baby), I'll do things such as organizing my personal stuff—including Katherine's photo album and her baby book—writing baby announcements, and packing my suitcase for the hospital.

I continue going to physical therapy two times a week. With the exception of stress from work, things are going well.

Fred, Katherine, and I are looking forward to our new baby. We all wonder if it will be a boy or a girl. Katherine's excited about being a "big sister." She goes to most of my [doctor] visits to hear her baby brother or sister's heartbeat. The look in her eyes is precious. We have so much to be thankful for!

On October 5, I tested positive for Group B Strep (GBS). Group B Strep, a bacterium, causes no harm in the vaginas of healthy women. However, it can cause a very serious infection in newborns, who can get it while passing through the vagina during birth. I took Amoxicillin three times a day until October 12, and then reduced it to once a day until my delivery. From October 2 until the day I gave birth, I recorded the abdominal cramping that I experienced. I was hoping that I could deliver this baby on my own, without Pitocin.

October 13: My last [doctor] visit was October 10. If I don't have our baby by Monday, October 17, I'm scheduled for an induction. I'm supposed to call the hospital at 7:30 A.M. to see if they have any obstetrics beds available. If they do, they expect me

there by 8:00 A.M. I'm glad that I don't have to wait any longer
than that (I'll be nine days past the due date). We're all so excited!
It's hard to believe that in four days (or sooner) we'll be holding
our new baby: Michael James or Holly Marie.

On Saturday, October 15, I started getting contractions at
5:30 A.M. I began to record each one at 7:45 A.M. I put stars by
the ones that were strong; a pattern developed, and the majority
of them became stronger. I phoned the doctor on call, and he
told me to come to the hospital when my contractions were five
to six minutes apart. The hospital was only two blocks from our
home. At 10:27 A.M., my back started hurting during contractions. At the time, I thought it was important to record the precise minute. I also kept track of other physical signs that led me
to believe that I would have our baby that day.

To help take my mind off the contractions, I went to my next-
door neighbor's to visit. I continued monitoring the contractions. They became closer together, and my back pain was more
intense with each one; I even had to stop talking during each
contraction. I went back home and told Fred it was time to go
to the hospital. We arrived there at noon.

The back pain during my contractions was becoming unbearable. At 1:45 P.M. my water broke. I was dilated 4–5 centimeters.
At 2:30 P.M. I told Fred that if I didn't get an epidural soon, I was
going to the nurses' station and insist on one. At 2:45 P.M. I
received the epidural and felt immediate relief. My contractions
were three minutes apart, which made it difficult for me to keep
still while the anesthesiologist was putting the epidural in (it's hard

to remain motionless and bend forward during an excruciating contraction). Concentration was imperative. This epidural was more effective than the one I had during my labor with Katherine.

At some point, I learned that my back pain was caused by my labor. The back of the baby's head was pressing against my sacrum, the rear boundary of the pelvis, causing intense pain during contractions. Although I felt better because of the epidural, we were anxious because the baby's heart rate decreased every time I had a contraction. During the delivery, we learned that the cord was wrapped around our baby's neck.

At 3:48 P.M. Holly Marie was born. She weighed 8 pounds 9 ounces and was 21 inches long. Holly required suctioning immediately. The neonatal nurse stabilized Holly and removed the meconium from her airway. Holly's first Apgar score (which rates the condition of a newborn on a scale of 0–10) was only a 1. Until the early 1950s, there was no standard way to quickly evaluate an infant's condition at birth. The Apgar score was developed by the late Dr. Virginia Apgar, former professor of anesthesiology at Columbia College of Physicians and Surgeons. The system, used routinely in hospitals, evaluates heart rate, respiratory effort, muscle tone, reflex irritability, and color at one minute and five minutes after birth. Most physicians believe the five-minute test tells more about baby's true health. Holly's subsequent scores were 7 and 9. We were relieved and thankful! After the neonatal nurse stabilized Holly, we were allowed to hold her for only a few minutes because she needed to be put on oxygen. I will always treasure holding her the first time. Our eyes locked and we had an immediate connection—she knew I was her mom. Fred and I immediately fell in love with our precious baby daughter.

Holly remained on oxygen throughout most of the night. She had to endure several blood tests, and she had to be monitored by a neonatologist for two days, but after that, all was well.

Chapter 8

Post-Pregnancy

After Katherine was born on the night of December 8, 1991, she remained in my hospital room with me for most of December 9. Even though I wanted her to sleep with me that night, I knew that I needed uninterrupted sleep (as much as you can get in a hospital with all the necessary monitoring), so it was in my best interest to have her sleep in the nursery.

December 10: On Monday, December 9, I got up at 7:00 A.M. I had had about two hours of sleep. Every muscle in my body ached. I went to sleep between 11:30 P.M. and midnight. I woke up and missed Katherine. I couldn't sleep from 1:30 to 2:30 A.M. I ended up spending most of the night with her. Katherine and I slept from 5:30 to 7:30 A.M. [Tuesday]. *Fred was here two times between 2:30 and 7:30 P.M.*

Prior to my going off medication, we decided that I would nurse our baby for as long as I could, before I had to go back on lithium. My perception was that I would be fully aware of when I should resume lithium. Boy, was I wrong.

It's very important to remember that while experiencing manic or depressive episodes, a person is quite caught up in the moment; logic and common sense often disappear. Trusting others and relying on them for feedback about restarting medication is vital.

While I was off lithium, it was helpful to describe my bipolar symptoms in my journal. If I didn't have the journal with me, I would write in my calendar. At times, however, I was not able to conceptualize my behavior. Going back and reviewing what I wrote was an important reference and a good reality check.

I also knew that my husband would let me know if he thought I should go back on lithium. Dr. Eerdmans told me to call her when my bipolar symptoms returned. (I address my personal thoughts on nursing and resuming medication after delivery in Chapter 10.)

Anyway, back to my first complete night after Katherine was born: Here I was in the hospital, trying to catch up on sleep. The night before I was induced, I slept for about three hours in the hospital. I was exhausted after fifteen and a half hours of rigorous labor and delivery (there's no way I'm rounding it down to fifteen hours) and had slept only two hours that night. Because of my lack of judgment, the next night, December 9, I slept less than three hours. Without even realizing it, I had set myself up for a manic or depressive episode. This is what happened.

Once I finally fell asleep, I woke up and kept thinking about Katherine. I missed her more than I ever thought possible, even though she was right down the hall, and I knew I'd see her in the morning. I tried to go back to sleep, but I was overwhelmed by my desire to be with her that very moment. So at 2:30 A.M., I walked to the nursery and asked if I could see Katherine. It was feeding time and the nurse asked if I wanted to breastfeed her in my room. I was happy because it would give me a chance to bond with her and practice nursing.

The nurse brought Katherine to my room, and we agreed that Katherine would return to the nursery when I was finished. I knew that I needed to sleep that night, but I was too wound up. I nursed her—it was a challenging but fulfilling experience. My love for Katherine was so intense. At 3:30 A.M., Katherine was back in the nursery, and I was looking forward to going to sleep. I was exhausted.

Within thirty minutes, half asleep, I heard Katherine crying. Sure enough, the crying became louder, because the nurse was bringing her to my room. Katherine had been crying for a while, and the nurse asked if I would try to calm her down. Of course I agreed. The nurse left, and Katherine and I were alone. I walked with her, rocked her, talked and sang to her, and nursed her again. I admit, I was at my threshold and had second thoughts about my previous decision to visit Katherine in the first place—I needed sleep.

Finally, about 5:30 A.M., Katherine fell asleep and I put her in her bassinette, rolled it next to my bed, and we both slept until 7:30 A.M.

Because sleep is so important for new mothers, especially those who are bipolar, I believe that keeping your baby in the nursery at night during your hospital stay is worth considering. It might be the last night or two for quite a while that you get uninterrupted sleep. Most likely, you'll feel more energized to spend quality time with your newborn in the morning.

December 10 [continued]: *I had a hectic day. I slept about two hours last night. I was busy every minute at the hospital (CPR and bathing classes for Katherine, learning how to nurse effectively, talking to Katherine's pediatrician, and preparing to go home). We left the hospital at 8:30 P.M. Katherine's pediatrician gave me some practical advice. He suggested that I prioritize my day in the following way:*

1. *Have to do: feed and take care of Katherine*

2. *Want to do: style my hair, do my nails, clean house*

3. *Ought to do: Don't count on getting this done—it's not important.*

Fred recalled the following:

The whole experience of Katherine's birth was one of the most cherished times of my life. Because I was older than many first-time fathers (forty-two), it was even more special. My brother and three sisters all have children whom I love, but Katherine, our first baby, gave me absolute joy! Kristin and I overcame several challenges, but beautiful Katherine was our greatest reward.

Before leaving the hospital, Fred, Katherine, and I had a memorable dinner together. The hospital treated us to a special farewell meal. Fred was both intrigued and mesmerized by Katherine. The love he had for her radiated from his face. He told me how proud he was of me during Katherine's birth. I felt so loved and appreciated, and occasionally I caught him looking at me with admiration. Going home for the first time with Katherine was an unbelievable experience.

On the way home, however, I thought about what we had recently been through with Katherine's birth. For the past few days, I had been in my own world, adjusting to our new baby. It was strange being outside the hospital; we had recently experienced a miracle, and now I felt as if everything else around me was "business as usual." Katherine, Fred, and I entered our home together for the first time. Our life as parents was now beginning!

The first four days at home with Katherine were enjoyable. I started filling in the Baby's First Year Sticker Calendar to help keep track of daily activities and, of course, Katherine's "firsts." For example, giving Katherine her first bath was challenging. Fred and I referred to a book that told us step-by-step how to bathe her. We soon realized that there was a lot more to it than we thought. Seeing her first smile warmed our hearts. We were so happy to have our precious daughter, Katherine Kay. However, the next nine weeks opened a world of challenges.

When Katherine was only seven days old, I developed mastitis (breast infection) from nursing. This experience, along with the clogged milk ducts that developed four weeks later, was extremely stressful. I relied on the information in *What to Expect When You're Expecting* (Murkoff, Eisenberg, & Hathaway, 2002). The La Leche League, the hospital where you delivered, breastfeeding support groups, and your own ob-gyn are also invaluable resources.

December 15: I have a temperature of 102.4 and feel as if I have the flu. My left breast has clogged milk ducts—I can't escape the pain.

We phoned the doctor on call, who told me that I had mastitis and prescribed Tegopen, an antibiotic. It was Sunday night, the closest open pharmacy was on the other side of town, and we were in the middle of a snowstorm. Fred picked up the Tegopen, and I began taking it late Sunday evening.

December 16: My mom spent the day with us. Nursing Katherine with my left breast gives me excruciating pain.

My mom called my aunt, who is a La Leche League consultant (the group provides advice and support for moms who breastfeed) and a mother of nine. She gave us the following tips for treating plugged milk ducts:

- Use a heating pad on the affected area.

- Nurse in alternating positions, such as a clutch hold (like holding a football), cradle, and lying down.

- Ice the affected area.

- Apply Bag Balm to the affected area. (This is a salve used for a cow's painful udder.) It can be found at many stores in the health and beauty sections and comes in a distinctive square green tin.

- Nurse every two to three hours.

The doctor on call also prescribed Nuprin (ibuprofen) every four hours for the pain.

December 16 [continued]: *My temperature has decreased to 100.2, but I still feel terrible.*

Then another problem developed.

December 17: I have consistent heavy bleeding [it came on suddenly, nine days after delivery]. *Fred called Dr. Hiemenga's office and described my symptoms. She prescribed Methergine to stop the bleeding.*

Fred and I were scared. At the time, we thought that I might go into shock or die as a result of losing so much blood. I realize that this might sound extreme, but that's how worried we were. I started taking Methergine every four hours, from 1:30 P.M. until 4:00 A.M. on December 19. I was also told to take Tylenol (acetaminophen) instead of ibuprofen for pain and to stay in bed.

It appeared that I was a likely candidate for postpartum hemorrhage. In *What to Expect When You're Expecting* (2002), the authors explain postpartum hemorrhage as follows:

Postpartum hemorrhage is heavy bleeding that is difficult to stem. It is a very serious but extremely uncommon complication.

And, when treated promptly, it is rarely the life-threatening situation it once was. Excessive bleeding may occur if the uterus is too relaxed and doesn't contract, due to a long, exhausting labor; a traumatic delivery; a uterus that was overdistended because of multiple births, a large baby, or excess amniotic fluid. . . . (page 525)

The doctor on call phoned me at 6:30 P.M. on December 17 to see how the Methergine was working and to summarize specific signs to look out for. If I was still bleeding in the morning, I was to call Dr. Hiemenga's office to schedule an ultrasound. This increased my stress level even more.

To help maintain some control during the mastitis and hemorrhaging, I kept records that summarized the following:

- The previously mentioned tips from my aunt about mastitis—that in itself was a lot to keep track of.

- A list of the times that I took my three medications. Example: Methergine and Tylenol, every four hours; Tegopen, every six hours.

On December 17 and 18, Fred stayed home from work to take care of Katherine and me. My mom stayed with us on Thursday, December 19, and Friday, December 20. Nursing Katherine started to get better on Thursday. My bleeding stopped completely on December 21, but I continued to tire easily. I kept detailed records until that morning.

December 24, Christmas Eve, was my first time out of the house since Katherine's birth. First I went out by myself to get my hair cut. I felt as if I had a sign on my forehead that said, "I just had a baby." It was good to get out; I felt independent. Later that evening, Fred, Katherine, and I went to church—our first outing as a family. By December 26, I started getting stronger. It was wonderful to get to know Katherine and to focus on her rather than on my health issues. The last week in December went smoothly.

The week of January 1, 1992, my lower back began to hurt. On January 9, I had an appointment at a pain clinic. By this time, I was at wits' end with the pain in my back. The doctor gave me a spinal block and an injection of Toradol, which is a nonsteroidal anti-inflammatory drug (NSAID). It didn't seem to help much. The lifting and bending involved in caring for a baby increased my back pain. On January 11, I started feeling sluggish and felt a sore throat coming on.

On January 13, my left breast started getting sore. Immediately I began nursing Katherine each time with my left breast, even though it hurt immensely. I also nursed her often. I didn't want to get another breast infection. By January 16, my left breast was red and hard, indicating that my milk ducts were plugged. I started applying heat and Bag Balm and recorded my nursing routine once again. My goal was to address this before it got worse.

My sore throat continued. I also had a runny nose, and my right ear began to hurt (my first earache—boy, does that hurt). I felt rundown and was not getting much sleep. On January 16 a doctor prescribed 25 milligrams (mg) of Dycill, an antibiotic, for my breast infection. On January 18, both ears hurt through-out the night. My right ear was plugged, and it was hard to hear. I felt terrible. In addition to all this, my back pain persisted.

January 20: Mom visited again. My back is getting worse. It hurts when I sit in a chair or recliner, even when I'm not holding Katherine.

January 21: This past week, I've had to hold Katherine during most of the day. My average day goes like this: I sit in the recliner downstairs [in our living room] *holding Katherine. I put her bouncy seat to the right of me, on a chair. Because I can't stand up while I'm holding her, I have to put her in the bouncy seat before getting up. This requires a lot of twisting. It's frustrating because I can't walk with Katherine, put her in her swing, or even lay her in her crib. I can't care for my own daughter, and I feel helpless and disheartened.*

January 13–17 was difficult for me on two distinct levels. The first was the physical aspect of my back problem. The repetitive twisting that took place exacerbated the pain. I had no idea that I had repeatedly broken several cardinal rules for having a healthy back, until I went to physical therapy on January 23. My therapy included weekly sessions in using proper body mechanics while lifting as well as during daily activities. It's always best to keep the object you are lifting (in this case, Katherine) close to you while lifting it. Twisting should be avoided. Use your legs, and avoid reaching and bending. My physical therapist also advised me to buy the book *Managing Back Pain* by Michael Melnik, Robin Saunders, and Duane Saunders (1989).

By this time Katherine weighed almost twelve pounds. Picture the steps I went through whenever I got up while I was alone. I held her more than a foot away from me when putting her in the bouncy seat, and each time I had to twist to the right. Ouch! I thought I was clever using this method, but the entire time I was making my back worse.

Weak abdominal muscles after surgery make you more susceptible to back injury. Start a postpartum exercise program, including abdominal strengthening, as soon as your ob-gyn gives his or her approval. Strong abdominal muscles help to support the back with all the added bending and lifting associated with a newborn. This will decrease your chances of a back injury.

My physical therapist gave me the following tips for my back (it probably doesn't surprise you that I wrote them down as she summarized them):

1. Pretend that a string is attached to your head from above. Stand and sit up straight.

2. Tighten your abdominal muscles—this tightens your abdomen and rear end muscles and flattens your lower back (similar to the pelvic tilt).

3. While picking something up (including your baby), follow these guidelines: Bend your knees, not your back; keep your back straight; do not bend forward at the waist; use the strength in your legs; keep your spine in line with your hips—don't twist.

4. Don't cross your legs while sitting.

The psychological ramifications of my back pain were also difficult. Every day seemed exactly the same. Fred would leave for work, and I would take care of Katherine while sitting in our recliner. Once he left, I felt isolated. I felt trapped in the recliner as well as in our house. Fred came home for lunch every day and came straight home after work. He was my lifeline. I looked forward to seeing him walk through our front door as never before. I don't know what I would have done without his support.

Fred said the following:

> Kristin's back problems created some new challenges for me. I knew she needed my ongoing support until she was physically able to care for Katherine. I altered my work schedule to be home at lunch, and reduced my running and workout routine. Taking care of Kristin and Katherine was my first priority. Everything else could wait.

January 23: Today at 11:00 A.M. I had an appointment with the doctor at the pain clinic. I can barely walk. It's a new challenge every time I have to get out of a chair or my bed. He says I have severe tendonitis of the sacroiliac [the joint between the top part of the pelvis and the fused bottom vertebrae] *area. He immediately prescribed a physical therapy evaluation. I have a 1:00 P.M. appointment today. My back is supposed to bend 117 degrees to touch my toes; my movement is limited to 17 degrees. I have limited movement in my sacroiliac area. I have a long way to go. Initial treatment includes hot packs, ultrasound, stretching, and ice packs. I've been getting severe lower back spasms.*

January 25: The back spasms on January 23 and 24 were excruciating! They come with no warning. As I became increasingly tense and agitated, they intensified. I could not sleep in my bed because I needed support for my back. I sat in the recliner downstairs with Fred by my side. I had constant spasms between midnight and 1:00 A.M. (I was shaking uncontrollably). The spasms were piercing. I felt guilty because I had trouble feeding Katherine. I couldn't even be near her. Hearing Katherine cry made me tremble and put my back in constant spasm. My back hurt so much, I wanted to go to the hospital by ambulance—and have them drug me to ease the pain. I slept no more than one to two hours. I could hardly walk.

On January 24 I was up by 5:00 A.M. I called Mom at 6:30 A.M. I was shaking horrendously, which magnified my spasms. I couldn't even tell her about the plan Fred and I had discussed that morning. Fred had to finish the conversation for me. Next to childbirth, this was the worst pain I had ever experienced.

Fred told my mom that we had decided I should go on pain medication to decrease the spasms. We knew that I would have to temporarily quit nursing Katherine while I was on this medication.

Fred and I had previously rented an electric breast pump (they are fast and easy to use), so I was prepared to pump milk regularly. My plan was to continue to produce milk and throw it away until I quit taking the medication and could safely nurse Katherine again. Reflecting on this now, I question our decision for me to return to nursing once the pain medication was out of my system. Given the unique circumstances, this would have been an ideal time for me to stop nursing and resume lithium. Katherine was seven weeks old.

January 25 [continued]: I called the doctor at the pain clinic and summarized my recent experience and proposed plan. He prescribed 800 mg of ibuprofen and 5 mg of Valium. I nursed Katherine and then started the medication at 9:30 A.M. Katherine will take formula until I go off the pain medication. I might even decide to stop nursing completely. She was fussy during her noontime feeding, which made me feel guilty and helpless. By dinnertime, Katherine started drinking the formula really well.

I had trouble walking and getting out of the recliner all day. Fred took the recliner upstairs to our room earlier this morning because I have difficulty going up and down stairs. The meds have taken the edge off the pain, and I can relax. Relaxing the muscles helps to keep the spasms under control. I have physical therapy at 5:45 P.M. Fred will drive me. I bought a lumbar support pillow to use while sitting. It helps to stabilize my back. My back seems to hurt the most after therapy. I slept like a rock during the night. What a blessing!

January 26: My back pain continues. Although the spasms have decreased, I still have to support my back against a wall when I sneeze to avoid severe pain. I have therapy at 10:00 A.M. I'm noticing lots of improvement. Fred has been terrific helping me get through this ordeal. Taking care of Katherine and me and doing the housework, laundry, and grocery shopping is a challenge for anyone. He stayed home from work Thursday and Friday to care for us. I slept well again. I'm sure the medications help.

I can't stress the importance of having a supportive partner.

Even if you don't have any physical difficulties after childbirth, adjusting to a newborn is challenging under ideal circumstances. Partners should make a special effort to be as helpful and available as possible.

January 26 [continued]: *The recliner is still upstairs. I'm improving, but I have a long way to go. Mom will be here tonight and tomorrow. I can't lift Katherine for at least one or two weeks, so I'm getting help next week.*

My mother made the following comments:

> Living so far away from my daughter and granddaughter was frustrating for me. We talked on the phone a lot during Katherine's first nine weeks as Kristin and Fred went from one crisis to another. New parents shouldn't have to deal with all these problems simultaneously. My plan before Katherine's birth was to be available but to let Kristin, Fred, and Katherine function alone together as a new family. Visiting overnight as I did on January 26 was actually easier for me because I was there doing things to help out. Caring for little Katherine was such a gift. Holding, rocking, bathing—I loved every minute of it, and I got to interact with Kristin even though she was immobile and miserable much of the time. Kristin's dad and I are so thankful for Fred—he's a one-in-a-million son-in-law.

Since I could not lift Katherine, Fred and I were fortunate to have various friends and family members to help us take care of her during the next five weeks while Fred was at work. A visiting nurse helped out a couple of days when we had scheduling

conflicts. Setting up this schedule took planning and organizing, but we didn't have a choice. My identity as a mom was
crumbling, and I had no idea how to get it back.

February 7–9, I went on a retreat with my mom. She had the
following to say:

> For several years, Kristin and I had enjoyed attending a church
> retreat together. Retreat weekend that winter was not what I had
> anticipated. Katherine was two months old, and usually new par-
> ents would have settled into a flexible routine by then. This was not
> the case at all. I was waiting at our usual retreat location when Fred
> dropped Kristin off. He and Katherine then traveled about an hour
> to spend the weekend at Fred's parents' home. This was another
> "first." Their family of three had never been apart.
>
> Along with bringing her suitcase, Kristin arrived with her fancy
> electric breast pump in its carrying case and various cushions and
> pillows to help ease her back pain. She was determined to resume
> breastfeeding when she no longer needed the prescription pain pills
> for her back. Her milk supply remained available as long as she
> pumped as needed (the milk was thrown away).
>
> While alone in our room, we came to the realization that enough
> is enough! Until then, breastfeeding had been such a priority; we
> had overlooked the fact that Kristin's hypomanic symptoms were
> escalating. It was time to call Dr. Eerdmans. Kristin had already
> been lithium free for a year. This is a good example of the benefit of
> "retreating" from an out-of-hand situation in order to take a more
> objective look at yourself.

Chapter 9

Peace of Mind—
Back on Medication

February 11, 1992: *During the weeks of January 27 and February 3, a number of people came to our house to help me take care of Katherine. My back is getting stronger, but I still can't stand up and hold Katherine when she's on my lap. It's totally aggravating. Today was the first day I didn't have help in the morning. A girl from my church comes to help me every day from 2:00 to 4:45 P.M.*

Over the weekend while at a retreat with my mom, we talked about my going back on lithium. I spoke to Dr. Eerdmans yesterday, and she agreed. I knew something was wrong when she asked me how it was being a mom. Immediately I felt overwhelmed. I told her I wished I was able to enjoy Katherine more—I feel so worried, isolated, and confused. Dr. Eerdmans told me to start taking lithium three times a day. [It had been nine weeks since Katherine was born.] *Even though it's only been twenty-four hours since I started taking it again, somehow I feel it working.*

For the past couple weeks I've been feeling especially isolated and anxious—as if my life is out of control. I love Katherine dearly, but it's so hard because I can't even hold her (except when I'm sitting down), rock her, or walk with her. In summary, I can't take care of her without someone else's assistance.

I miss spending time with Fred. I feel as if I'm drowning in guilt and remorse because I haven't been contributing much. In addition to caring for Katherine and me, he takes care of the house. Sometimes I just want my "old life" back. That's when I realized that I do need to go back on lithium. It's as if my emotions have been tossed into a blender. My hypomanic symptoms are taking over. I'm desperate to feel peace again.

Fred added the following comments:

> When Kristin decided to go back on lithium, I supported her decision wholeheartedly. Kristin's goal was to breastfeed for three months, but her physical problems were taking over her thoughts and emotions. I knew she felt guilty because she couldn't help with the household chores and take better care of Katherine, but to me that was no big deal. It was more important for her to rest, which at that point was impossible without lithium. Breastfeeding for seven weeks was a good start for Katherine; now it's time for Kristin to get healthy.

February 12 [two days after I resumed lithium]: *Hindsight is 20/20. Here are some additional warning signs that I had been experiencing for the past couple weeks that prove it was time for me to go back on lithium:*

1. *I had several talks with Fred about possibly having only one child. I kept feeling as if I had to justify why I thought that might be best. Fred has never pressured me about having a second baby, but the topic was constantly on my mind.*

2. *I would wake up in the middle of the night and not be able to get back to sleep, worrying about all kinds of things.*

3. *Everything was a big deal.*

4. *I didn't want to eat as much as I usually do.* [That's a shocker—now we know something's wrong.]

5. *I wanted to stay in bed in the morning because it felt safe.*

I didn't write anything in my pregnancy journal or calendar about the unnerving realization that I could not nurse Katherine again. I was so overwhelmed by my emotions that I needed to do whatever was necessary to feel good again. I used my breast pump sporadically to relieve some of the pressure. Knowing that my breastfeeding days were over, I didn't want to stimulate milk production.

On February 21, I went to a two-hour post-pregnancy support group. I enjoyed meeting other moms who had recently had babies. The group facilitator encouraged us to talk about what we considered important. It was fun to watch Katherine interact with other babies. A woman who had a baby Katherine's age lived one block from me. This was the beginning of a friendship. Our relationship was helpful for us as new moms and for our girls.

I'm glad I kept track of everyday events by using the Baby's First Year Sticker Calendar. It was a great way of remembering the positive things about this pregnancy. I'd recommend it to any new mom—bipolar or not. I was able to relive the cherished memories and special "firsts" that would otherwise have been a blur. Without it, I would have focused on the tough times during Katherine's first two months rather than on the wonderful times I'll always treasure. I would have forgotten her first smile, her first outing, her first coos, her first time standing (with help), and the first time she saw her grandparents and other relatives. Now we can remember how she spent her days that entire first year.

Filling in the calendar regularly was manageable. Even today, Katherine and I occasionally look at it together. The stickers and comments evoke positive memories of her babyhood. I also had a baby book for Katherine, but just thinking about completing it those first few months was overwhelming. Once I felt better, I transferred the special memories to it. The details of Katherine's first year are precious and irreplaceable.

Three things helped me to get back on track after Katherine's birth. First, resuming lithium helped me to feel more in control. I'm fortunate to have a chemical imbalance that can be controlled with medication and talk therapy. Second, Fred provided stability in my life. He was a ray of sunshine, even if my day was stormy. Fred has always been my anchor. The third thing that helped was physical therapy.

Fred noted the following:

It felt as if another marathon had been completed once Kristin finished physical therapy. She was physically stronger, and we were even able to travel to Colorado so I could enjoy spring skiing. For Kristin, it was a wonderful change of scenery. After our trip the weather was warmer, so we could take Katherine for walks in our neighborhood. Kristin was healthy, and her perspective and outlook were transformed. We had reached the point where we could have a normal life with a four-month-old daughter, who was our shining star.

It's hard to have peace of mind when you're constantly in pain. My last day of physical therapy was April 9, 1992. I was ready to start exercising on my own (using good judgment, of course). Had I not had so many post-pregnancy complications, I would have started sooner.

Because of the significant physical and emotional health benefits that exercise provides (especially for bipolars), I believe that the following questions, from the article "Postpartum Exercise: Is Your Body Ready?" (www.babycenter.com) are important to consider. After giving birth, always talk with your doctor before exercising.

How soon after delivery can I start exercising? The American College of Obstetricians and Gynecologists say it's okay to gradually resume exercising when you feel up to it. But your doctor or midwife may ask you to wait until your six-week postpartum checkup so she can see how you're doing first.

Generally, if you exercised throughout your pregnancy and had a normal vaginal delivery, you can safely perform your pregnancy workout—or at least light exercise, such as walking, modified push-ups, and stretching—within days of giving birth. After your first postpartum week, a slow to moderate 30-minute walk three times a week is fine. As you regain strength, you can increase the length or number of walks.

If you had a c-section, expect to wait about six to eight weeks to exercise. However, walking at an easy pace is encouraged because it promotes healing and helps prevent complications such as blood clots.

If you weren't active during your pregnancy, or tapered off your fitness routine as the weeks went on, start slow and check with your doctor or midwife before you begin exercising.

In any case, remember that your joints and ligaments will still be loose for about three to five months, so watch your step to avoid spills. If you want to take an exercise class, try to find one taught by a postpartum exercise specialist or go for a low-impact class focused on toning stretching. Many YMCA's, recreation centers, gyms, and yoga studios offer exercise class for new moms.

Exercise is good for you, but in the first few months after you give birth, don't overdo it. Your body needs time to heal, and you need time to adjust to your new role and to care for and bond with your baby.

Do I need to be careful of my abdominal muscles? Most women develop a gap in their abdominal muscles as their belly expands during pregnancy and labor. It takes approximately four to eight weeks after giving birth for this gap to close.

If you start doing abdominal exercises before the gap closes, you risk injuring those muscles—so make sure your belly is ready before you start . . .

Will exercise affect my ability to breastfeed? No, it won't. Even vigorous exercise doesn't significantly affect the amount or composition of your breast milk. But you'll want to avoid exercises that make your breasts sore or tender. Wear a supportive sports bra while working out, and try to nurse your baby before you exercise so your breasts won't feel uncomfortably full.

Are there any physical signs that I might be trying to do too much too soon? Too much physical activity during the first few weeks after delivery can cause your vaginal flow, called lochia, to become pink or red and to flow more heavily. This is a signal to slow down. Notify your doctor or midwife if vaginal bleeding or lochia restarts after you thought it had stopped or if you experience any pain when you exercise.

What's the best way to lose weight after giving birth? The best way to start dropping those pregnancy pounds is to do some form of aerobic exercise to get your heart rate up, such as brisk walking, swimming, running, or biking.

But wait at least six weeks—and preferably a few months—before you actively try to slim down. And don't aim to lose more that a pound per week, especially if you're breastfeeding.

Starting a diet too soon after giving birth can affect your mood and energy level, as well as your milk supply. If you're patient and give your body time to do its work, you may be surprised at how much weight you lose naturally.

That concludes my post-pregnancy experiences with Katherine. Fred and I had many difficult times, but we worked together and have a wonderful daughter who completes our lives.

Post-Pregnancy Experiences with My Second Child

My post-pregnancy experience with Holly was a breeze compared to what I went through with Katherine. Holly was on oxygen in the nursery until the morning after she was born, so that's where we spent time with her. I felt energized and cheerful immediately after Holly was born. What a contrast from how I felt after Katherine's birth! My mom and dad brought Katherine (who was almost three) to the hospital to meet her baby sister as soon as they heard the news.

Katherine wasn't sure what was happening. As soon as she entered my room, she crawled into bed with me. It started out as a hug, and before I knew it, she was under the covers with me. I remember thinking, "Easy does it, I just had a baby." We told her how much we loved her and focused on how special it was to be a big sister. I was hungry for a submarine sandwich, so my dad and Fred went out and got subs for all of us. We had fun celebrating Holly's birth.

My mom made the following observations:

> After Holly was born, I couldn't help but think that this was Kristin and Fred's reward after all they had gone through last time.

Kristin looked terrific right after delivery. We had a good time hanging out in her hospital room. I immediately looked forward to future visits with Kristin, Fred, and my two granddaughters.

On October 16, the day after Holly was born, the neonatologist examined Holly and discussed her delivery with us. She continued to require monitoring but was doing well. Fred was in awe of his baby girl—we both were. Watching him look at Holly gave me a sense of inner peace. We had quite a few visitors, and Holly spent a lot of time in my room. She was precious. It was hard to believe that I felt so good so soon—physically and mentally. On Monday, October 17, Holly and I came home from the hospital. She was two days old.

Fred stayed home from work October 17–21 to spend time with Holly, Katherine, and me. We set this time aside to adjust to our new family. Katherine went to day care Tuesday through Thursday. Fred and I continued to focus on the importance of Katherine's role as the big sister. We encouraged her to help us care for Holly. Our goal was for Katherine to feel included and loved. Katherine showed us how much she loved baby Holly. Her face lit up like fireworks when they were together. The seeds for a sisterly bond were sprouting.

However, there was still one problem. Katherine wasn't even three and didn't understand bipolar disorder. (Then again, what kid does?) I chose to nurse Holly, so therefore I would continue to be without my medication. If I had to struggle to control my mind, how could I care for Katherine and Holly?

Prior to conception, while I was still on lithium, Fred and I agreed that I would nurse Holly only until it was necessary for me to restart medication. We learned so much from the complications I had while nursing Katherine. For example, I would stop nursing and start taking lithium once my bipolar symptoms returned or if I had too much stress. It sounds obvious, but it's important to rethink plans that have major consequences. Doing this was comforting.

My intention was to abide by our agreement, even if my bipolar symptoms told me to do otherwise. If you are considering nursing, make sure to write down your plan before medication changes. Once your plan is in place, stick to it.

On October 19 my milk started coming—ouch! I felt depressed and overwhelmed. I knew that I should be happy because everything was going smoothly. I didn't understand why I felt like crying. I figured this must be the baby blues I had read about—it felt so real. At that time I chose not to dwell on it, hoping it would pass, which it did.

The next day, I noticed a lump the size of a grape under my arm. I knew I had a plugged milk duct. By the next day it had spread, and the pain grew worse. I immediately started the treatment for plugged milk ducts that I summarized in the previous chapter, and I made sure I got plenty of rest.

By October 22, I started feeling better—relief at last. I fed Holly breast milk from a bottle for the first time—Fred and I decided that bottle-feeding Holly once a day would help to prepare her for the imminent weaning process. We learned that she took a bottle best after her afternoon nap because she woke up ravenously hungry. We also planned to give her a bottle when I was out and about. Having the freedom to pump breast milk for Holly and to occasionally leave the house without her was reassuring. It helped me to maintain my independence.

The evening of October 22, Fred, Katherine, Holly, and I had our first family outing: We went to dinner. Holly slept through the meal, and we looked at her constantly (as if she were a new baby or something)! It felt terrific to be back in the mainstream of life.

My mom visited again October 23–25. She was helpful and supportive. We had so much fun together (and still do). On October 25, Mom, Holly, and I went shopping and out to lunch while Katherine was in day care. It was a magical day. I felt wonderful, and Holly was beginning to show her personality. I had an enjoyable week.

On November 2, Holly and I went to Challenges, the support group for women at my church. I had attended the group regularly prior to Holly's birth, and it felt good to start going again and get out of the house. I continued to build relationships there. Getting Holly and me ready by 9:30 A.M. was a challenge. Caring for a newborn is an all-encompassing responsibility. It is, however, important to make time for the activities that are rewarding.

I was diligent about completing a Baby's First Year Sticker Calendar for Holly. Just as I did for Katherine, I eventually transferred some of the "firsts" to Holly's baby book. It's interesting to see how her personality evolved. Holly now enjoys reminiscing about the things she did as a baby. I will always treasure her calendar and baby book. Fred might not appreciate the keepsakes the same way I do, but he gets a kick out of looking at them. The calendar also helped me to track how I was adjusting to our second baby.

Life in the Finn house was going smoothly until November 8. That's when I found out that our new sectional would be delivered two days later. I was excited because we would be able to start spending time in our newly finished family room. At dinner, Fred told me I was "wound up"—I was talking nonstop. In retrospect I agreed, but at that time I had no idea I would soon be out of control. I was concentrating on a mission that I planned to accomplish the next day.

My mission was to get ready for the delivery of the sectional. The sofa and the loveseat that we had upstairs in the living room would be moved down to the family room that evening. I cleaned and prepared the family room. I also organized all of Katherine's books and toys and took most of them to the family room, where we planned to hang out. Holly was only three and a half weeks old—physically and mentally I felt like the Energizer bunny. I described my behavior in my calendar as being "driven."

Fred noted the following:

> Kristin was wound up about the arrival of our new sectional for
> the living room. After building our house, the family room on the
> lower level was empty. She was on a mission to have everything

ready for the new layout. I had to tell her constantly to slow down and take it easy—it had only been three and a half weeks since Holly was born. However, when Kristin got into one of those moods, there was no stopping her. Rearranging furniture might sound ho-hum to many people, but the completion of our family room seemed like the most important thing in the world to her.

Even now, after all these years and experiences we've had together, when she gets on a mission to finish a task, I have to remind her to stop working, relax, and do something else for a while. It will be there when she returns.

In my experience, when mania takes over, everything else becomes invisible. It consumes me, and my objective is to accomplish whatever mission I perceive is important at the time. The bursts of energy are incredible. The downside is that agitation often accompanies mania if things don't go exactly as planned.

For example, on November 10, as I was waiting for our sectional to arrive, I received a phone call that it could not be delivered until the following day. You would have thought my world was coming to an end. I was overly disappointed and frustrated. I was counting on spending time in our new family room that evening. I know it shouldn't have been such a big deal, but to me it was. I overreacted to a minor situation that was out of my control. The next day proved to be the beginning of a new chapter in my life. Unfortunately, it was a nightmare getting there.

Later that same day, my mom and dad came to visit for a couple days. Katherine was in day care and Mom, Holly, and I went out for lunch. I vividly remember the following experience in detail. At the restaurant, my mind was racing uncontrollably. I felt very anxious. When my mom left the table to use the restroom, I knew that I did not want to be alone with my thoughts. They were coming at me so fast that I had to find a way to organize and understand them. I took my organizer out and wrote the following:

November 10, 1994: I think I have to go back on lithium. My mind is racing. When I'm having a conversation with someone, I can focus on what they're saying if I force myself to listen, but my mind thinks about several other things, like sidebars. It's as if I'm having endless conversations with myself that relate to the topic.

The following are my symptoms, or what I'm feeling, when my mind is racing:

- *At night when I try to sleep, even though I'm exhausted, it feels as if my mind is a separate entity. I want to sleep, but my mind won't stop thinking.*

- *Everything I do is very calculated—I want to be extremely precise.*

- *I feel guilty about having to go back on lithium because I know that breastfeeding is best for Holly.*

I realize that my decision to wean Holly is best for her, Fred, and Katherine. I know it's tough to live with me when I'm like this. It's

difficult for me, too. I feel imprisoned by this chemical imbalance. I
want to be able to control my racing mind, but I'm having such a
hard time without medication.

I believe that I would have crawled out of my skin had I not
expressed those feelings on paper during the few minutes that
my mom was gone. For me, being alone when my mind is racing is torture. Holly was asleep, so I couldn't interact with her.
When my mom returned, I told her how I was feeling. There was
no doubt that it was time for me to go back on lithium. I called
Dr. Eerdmans right away, and we played phone tag until later
that evening. Even though I knew I was skyrocketing out of control and needed to slow down, nothing could have stopped me
from keeping our 6:10 P.M. appointment to have Katherine and
Holly's Christmas picture taken.

Fred, Katherine, Holly, my mom, and I arrived at the crowded
photo studio at 6:10 sharp. The entire photo experience was a
blur to me. Throw in the confusion and noise you'd find at many
studios close to a holiday, and imagine how that fueled my
mania. There was the long wait after arrival, followed by the
picture taking and selection process. Fred and I were tense and
anxious. He later told me that I insisted on keeping this
appointment and that any attempt to stop me would have been
ignored. He was right! Because the photographers were running
behind, he even asked if I would reschedule once we were there.
Of course I emphatically said, "No!" Fred's insistence would only
have exacerbated my compulsion to get the Christmas picture
taken that evening.

Fred commented as follows:

The appointment was an absolute nightmare. Our time slot was for 6:10 P.M., but it was well after 7:00 before we began the process. I wanted to reschedule and leave, but there was no way Kristin would agree. She wanted it done that night, no exceptions!

Her behavior was agitated—almost bizarre. She was practically directing the photographer on how to do his job, how to pose the girls, and what background was best. She was talking nonstop, and I couldn't get her to calm down. I wanted to get this session over with as soon as possible to get away from the chaos. Afterward, Kristin, her mother, and I talked about her restarting lithium. It was so obvious to us that she was out of control.

Mom added the following:

From past experience, I knew that Kristin's bipolar symptoms would return. Being with her in the restaurant and that evening at the photo session left no doubt that it was time to call Dr. Eerdmans. I felt my role was to stay calm and be supportive. To say I was relieved and very tired when the day was over is an understatement.

Once we got home, I updated Dr. Eerdmans about my turbulent behavior. She agreed that I should resume lithium immediately. Because she truly understood what I had been going through, it was a relief talking with her about my feelings. I felt as if I had my own way of viewing the world, and Dr. Eerdmans had always connected with me. I would also have benefited from the empathy and encouragement of a bipolar support group.

After my conversation with Dr. Eerdmans, I had the permission I needed to restart lithium. I was comforted, knowing that I would soon experience a quiet and peaceful mind.

It's important for me to explain what I mean by getting "permission" from Dr. Eerdmans to go back on medication. Even though I knew it was best for my family and me, I felt guilty that I had to stop nursing Holly. She loved to nurse, and it was so hard taking that away from her. I was reassured that Dr. Eerdmans knew what I had been experiencing and that she agreed the time was right.

After talking with Dr. Eerdmans, I summarized the conversation for Fred and my parents. I went to our new family room (yes, the sectional was delivered that day) and nursed Holly for the last time. I felt a void knowing that this was the last time I would ever experience that special closeness (my perception was my reality). I valued every minute. Does this sound peculiar coming from someone who had some agonizing experiences while nursing her first child? Sometimes it's hard to explain why we feel the way we do. Perhaps it was because the choice to continue was not an option. Intellectually, I knew it was the right decision.

I couldn't wait to experience tranquility and control once lithium began working. Recall the volatile and turbulent scenarios that I experienced without lithium. Then picture me with control, peace of mind, and contentment. The latter was within reach, and it felt as if a weight had been lifted from my shoulders. That evening, nearly four weeks after Holly's birth, I confidently took lithium.

Holly took three days to adjust to drinking formula. The second day, in the evening, we switched her to a soy formula, and her fussiness decreased. Discontinuing nursing abruptly was physically painful, but I realized that it would be temporary. The next day I used the breast pump three times (for three to five minutes each), which decreased the engorgement. I limited the pumping to release the pressure without producing more milk. For pain I took 800 milligrams (mg) of ibuprofen and 325 mg of acetaminophen. If you have to start medication immediately, you might want to contact a lactation consultant to help you with the process of cold-turkey weaning.

In less than a week, the lithium started working, and I felt in control of my mind again, rather than it controlling me. I knew that I would experience ups and downs, as most people do, but they wouldn't be exaggerated. Holly was an expressive baby and smiled a lot. Katherine adapted to having a baby sister and often showed her love for Holly. Sometimes we even had to remind Katherine to be gentler when playing with her new sister. Fred and I were eager to begin another chapter in our lives with two daughters.

SUMMARY

Keep in mind the following helpful advice for managing a healthy post-pregnancy:

- While you are in the hospital, have your baby sleep in the nursery during the night; adequate rest is so important.

- If you choose to nurse, follow a prewritten plan that describes when you should make medication changes. Trust your partner and support team as you implement this plan.

- Follow the instructions given to prevent complications.

- Establish and maintain contact with a lactation consultant.

- Continue to monitor your feelings and bipolar symptoms by writing them down.

- Have realistic expectations for each day—prioritize.

- If you did not make medication changes after delivery, call your doctor at the first sign of bipolar or postpartum depression symptoms.

- Trust the feedback from your support team.

- Begin taking your medication as prescribed.

- Join a post-pregnancy or postpartum depression support group.

- Rely on your partner for ongoing support.

- Talk with your doctor about resuming or starting an exercise program.

Most of all, enjoy your new baby! It's also important to feel emotionally stable and secure once your baby is born. Dr. Eerdmans discusses this more in Appendix C.

Chapter 10

Looking Back:
If I Had Only Known...

"Hindsight is 20/20" is an appropriate cliché to describe this chapter. During both pregnancies, the way I handled a number of issues became evident after the fact. I'm going to share some of those reflections with you.

The Importance of Bipolar Disorder Education

Having a clear understanding of bipolar disorder and its ramifications is crucial. Prior to our decision to have children, my only perspective on this chemical imbalance was my own personal experience. Sheer determination and support from family, physicians, and friends helped me through the challenging times. My coping skills would have been better had I been more familiar with bipolar disorder.

In January 2004, I attended my first bipolar disorder seminar. It was offered through Cross Country Education of Nashville, Tennessee. Attendees included mental health professionals, nurses, marriage and family therapists, alcohol and drug counselors, and case managers. I went with a friend who is a school counselor. The name of the seminar was "Bipolar: A New Slant on the Disorder." It was written and presented by a psychologist named Jay Carter, whose insights you've read throughout this book.

I strongly encourage anyone who is bipolar to attend a seminar to learn more about diagnosis, treatment, and management. Supporters can benefit from this information as well. I found it fascinating. Dr. Carter's seminar validated me in many ways—I learned more about my behavior both on and off medication. He also gave explanations about my behavior before my bipolar diagnosis. It was cathartic. It took every ounce of control not to stand up and shout, "I can relate precisely to what you're saying!"

One of the most fascinating concepts he described, in my opinion, was how the prefrontal lobe of the brain works. Our executive functions (judgment, conscience, and awareness of the bigger picture) are found in the prefrontal lobe. Bipolars who are manic have very little activity in the prefrontal lobe. Since they have difficulty visualizing their actions and behaviors, they have trouble predicting them. Imagine how terrifying it would be to go off medication that helps to control your judgment, conscience, and awareness.

I tried to maintain my prefrontal lobe functions by being aware of my manic and depressive symptoms. I did this by recording my previous bipolar symptoms in a pregnancy journal. It helped me to identify the behaviors I wanted to avoid. From past experience, I knew that once I was off lithium, there would be times when I wouldn't be able to take a step back to observe and control my actions. This list of behaviors acted as my prefrontal lobe. It was a preventative way to monitor myself.

In Chapter 4, I explained how I tried to maintain my prefrontal lobe functions by writing out a list of guidelines. I clung to those points during this unpredictable time. I trained myself to concentrate and focus during all conversations. The first part of the list gave me a basic road map to follow; this was a list of my own personal rules. Referring to these points helped me to curb my negative behaviors.

Knowing that I would lack self-awareness, I also listed situations that were common even while I was taking medication. This kept me from being too hard on myself during these frequent occurrences. Years ago I consciously learned how to adapt to the way my mind works. Medication significantly decreased my bipolar symptoms, but I still needed to constantly scrutinize what I said and did.

Over many years I've learned to monitor my behavior by using ongoing checks and balances. Even when I'm taking medication, my mind works so fast that I'm usually thinking ahead. I've trained myself to listen effectively, think before I talk, and stay focused. It's unsettling to me if I'm talking with someone who goes off on an unrelated tangent before finishing the subject we were originally discussing. After I listen to such people complete their new thought or idea (which is often difficult), I try to bring the conversation back to our uncompleted topic. My goal was to do my best to focus and concentrate. I was determined to maintain self-control.

Your partner, family, and friends can also substitute for your prefrontal lobe. The references at the end of this book can help them to understand bipolar disorder. The more familiar they become with this subject, the more effectively they'll help you to maintain your judgment, consciousness, and awareness. In addition to their support, writing in a pregnancy journal will help to solidify your prefrontal lobe functions when you feel them slipping away. Three examples follow:

1. Fred consistently helped me to monitor my prefrontal lobe. I would ask if he thought I was talking too much or working excessively. Whom am I trying to kid? He regularly told me when I was working too much. He frequently encouraged me to slow down and relax. When I would get so wrapped up in the task at hand, it was hard to see myself and respond appropriately. After asking for Fred's opinion, I usually followed his advice. I trusted and respected him. During the period I was off medication, Fred became my prefrontal lobe because he was kind and caring yet firm. I know I would have responded negatively if he had been condescending and bossy. Keep this in mind, supporters!

2. I regularly asked my coworker to provide me with insight

about my personal and professional behavior. It gave me confidence and comfort when my own judgment had escaped me.

3. I used a pregnancy journal to help monitor my poor judgment. I concluded that long work hours, loss of sleep, my racing mind, and a compulsion to continually be productive go hand in hand. Writing (self-talk) was a way of reeling myself in, thus minimizing these manic symptoms.

The Importance of Sleep

Loss of sleep often fuels bipolar episodes. When mania takes over, you feel as if you need very little sleep. Besides that, it's extremely hard to quiet your mind so that you *can* sleep. Mania has made me feel excessively energized, motivated, and wired. The article "How to Get a Better Night's Sleep" (www.sleepless inamerica.org) provides the following tips:

- **Go to bed and wake up at the same time each day.** Getting your body used to a schedule can help regulate your sleep cycle.

- **Avoid sleeping in on weekends** to keep your schedule consistent and to make it easier to wake up on Mondays.

- **Relax before bedtime.** Set aside some time before bed to do things that relax you. A warm bath, reading, or listening to soft music . . . can help you unwind from the day.

- **Make a to-do-tomorrow list** if it bothers you to leave work undone at the end of the day.

- **Use natural or artificial light to help you.** Avoid bright lights before going to sleep. Wake up with the sun if possible. Spend some time in natural sunlight (not necessarily direct) during waking hours. If you can't wake up with the sun, turn bright lights on when you get up.

- **Get active early.** Try to exercise or do some type of physical activity for 20 to 30 minutes each day. But don't do it too close to bedtime. Three to six hours before going to bed is ideal.

- **Do something.** Don't lie in bed awake. This can make you anxious and worsen insomnia. Read or do another quiet activity until you feel tired.

- **Keep temperatures constant.** If the temperature in your bedroom is too hot or too cold, it could disrupt your sleep.

- **Keep your room dark.** Put up heavier blinds or use a sleep mask.

- **White noise,** such as radio static or the noise from a fan, helps some people sleep, especially if they are bothered by noises (such as traffic outside) that they can't control. Earplugs may also be helpful. . . .

- **When worries come to mind,** push them out by repeating a phrase in your mind like, "Not now, I'm resting/sleeping."

Join a Bipolar Support Group

Before making any changes in your medication, join a bipolar support group. I wish I had. My January 14, 1994, diary excerpt, found in Chapter 4, describes how a support group would have helped me. I felt agitated and isolated—I desperately needed to share my feelings, and I craved empathy and support from somebody who would have understood my circumstances.

The Depression and Bipolar Support Alliance (DBSA) is an excellent option (see the References for contact information). It is one of the nation's leading patient-directed organizations and focuses on the most prevalent mental illnesses: depression and bipolar disorder. DBSA support groups provide the kind of sharing and caring that is crucial for a lifetime of wellness. The groups do the following:

- Give you the opportunity to reach out to others and benefit from the experience of those who have "been there."

- Motivate you to follow your treatment plan.

- Help you to understand that a mood disorder does not define who you are.

- Help you to rediscover the strengths and the sense of humor that you thought you might have lost.

- Provide a forum for mutual acceptance, understanding, and self-discovery.

Support groups are not a substitute for professional care. DBSA chapters and support groups do not endorse or recommend the use of any specific treatment or medication. For such advice, you should consult your physician and/or mental health professional. The DBSA website (www.dbsalliance.org) can help you to find the DBSA chapter nearest you.

The National Alliance on Mental Health Illness (NAMI) is another organization that provides support, education, and advocacy. You'll find a wealth of information on their website (www.nami.org). It's also a good place to find a support group in your area.

The Importance of a Structured Career

Ideally, while you are off medication, your career should be well structured and consistent so that you can maintain control over this part of your life. For example, as I mentioned in Chapter 4, it was frustrating for me to work as a trade show marketing consultant, and I often felt as if I had no control. I worked far too much with very little to show for it. Despite my efficiency and diligence, the lack of control and accomplishment increased my stress level.

Listen to Your Body, Intuition, and Support Network

Once again I want to emphasize the importance of keeping a pregnancy journal to help monitor and manage your bipolar symptoms. In my journal entry of September 29, 1994 (see

Chapter 7), I mention that the only time my mind was racing and that I noticed manic behavior was when my dad and I had appointments. I vividly remember feeling driven and wired that day. I wasn't able to change my behavior—my prefrontal lobe functions had vanished. I should have canceled my 5:00 and 6:30 P.M. appointments or asked my dad to go on them without me. If Fred or my dad had suggested that I reschedule those appointments, I'm certain I would have said with conviction, "No, I'll be fine."

This stress probably caused my Braxton Hicks contractions, which were so strong that I became exhausted. Fortunately, I was close to my due date and was planning to stop working anyway. Otherwise, it would have been necessary to work fewer hours or stop completely. Who knows if I could have lived with that decision?

It's worth repeating that since it's hard to see yourself during manic or even hypomanic phases, you need to trust others to compensate for your impaired judgment. That's why it's so important for your partner, family, and friends to be familiar with bipolar signs and symptoms. Take their advice when you're having symptoms.

Prior to making any medication changes, write the following statement in your pregnancy journal: "I will listen to those in my support network for their input when my judgment is on hold."

My Personal Thoughts About Breastfeeding

I believe that my post-pregnancy experience with Katherine would have been healthier and more enjoyable had I bottle-fed her. Looking back, I wish I had resumed lithium right after Katherine was born.

Because I had made the decision to breastfeed, the ideal time to restart lithium would have been after starting on pain medication for my back. Feeling good mentally during that time would have made a big difference in my recovery. Why didn't I give myself permission to permanently wean Katherine? Poor judgment made me plan to resume nursing when the pain medication was out of my system. I simply was not thinking clearly.

Each breastfeeding experience is unique. I did much better nursing Holly. Shortly after I began having hypomanic symptoms, I resumed lithium and started bottle-feeding her. Both Holly and Katherine adjusted well to their abrupt weaning. If you decide to breastfeed, make sure you follow a written plan such as the one found in Chapter 2.

Join a Postpartum Support Group

Because bipolar women have a higher incidence of postpartum mania or depression, it's important to join a support group. Contact local hospitals for options. You can also contact Postpartum Support International (PSI) (see References for contact information). PSI was founded in 1987 to eliminate denial

and ignorance of emotional problems related to childbirth. Its
website (www.postpartum.net) has the following information:

Have you recently given birth? Are you feeling exhausted, anxious, depressed, or just not yourself? If you are—you are not alone.
Many women are not prepared for the wide range of emotions they
may experience after childbirth. They often feel sadness, anger,
anxiety, or a sense of inadequacy.

These feelings may vary in frequency and intensity, but are col-
lectively known as postpartum mood disorders. Help and support
is an important part of getting back to feeling like yourself again.
The important thing to remember is that the symptoms are temporary and treatable with skilled professional care and social support.
Whether you think you are depressed or just want more information, PSI is here to help.

I met with the Michigan coordinator for PSI. I was extremely
impressed with the pertinent information and support materials
that she shared with me. She has also started a postpartum
depression support group. Take advantage of these special professionals who are so giving and caring.

Additional sources are listed in the Websites section of the
References at the end of this book.

Dads need help, too. It's important for spouses or partners
to recognize the symptoms of postpartum depression so they
can provide encouragement to seek help. Many times they're
the first to identify this behavior. How can a new dad identify
something if he doesn't know what to look for? One of the

resources available to assist fathers is an outreach project supported by PSI; its website (www.postpartumdads.org) will
help dads and other family members by providing firsthand
information and guidance through the postpartum depression
experience.

Make the decision to take advantage of professional guidance
and support during this potentially turbulent time. It's best to
decide which postpartum depression support group to join
before making any medication changes. While you are busily
caring for your newborn baby, make it a priority to care for
yourself as well.

The next section of this chapter is written by Dr. Carter. He
discusses how his bipolar mother "borrowed" his prefrontal lobe.
It's important that supporters learn how to develop this skill. He
also addresses the prejudice and ignorance in our society about
bipolar disorder. The first time I read it, I knew I had an advocate in my corner. It even made me proud to be bipolar.

Doctor's Note

BY JAY CARTER, PsyD, DABPS

As I look back at my own life, I realize that my mother would borrow my prefrontal lobe when hers was dim. It was a good thing; she taught me how to use it. She taught me how to see the bigger picture, and she had faith and trust in a higher power. Her faith got her through some trying times.

Kristin was able to surrender her dysfunction when she was off medication. That is hard for someone who has had to try to exercise *more* control over herself than others. People who are bipolar have to exercise heavy-duty control over their moods and emotions, and it is done, sometimes, in quiet desperation. Surrender doesn't mean giving up; it means recognizing that assistance is needed. My mother was a brilliant woman who normally had a lot of common sense. When she was manic (I now realize), she would lose context. I remember that one time a man said something to her jokingly, and she took it literally. She turned to me and said angrily, "Did you hear what he said to me!?" I said, "He didn't mean it *that* way, Mom." She said, "Are you sure?" I said, "Yes." She surrendered that incident to me, trusting that I could see more clearly than she could at that moment.

I realize all this now in hindsight. I certainly didn't understand it back then.

I am surprised at how much prejudice there is in our society about bipolar disorder. First of all, it's not a *mental* illness; it is genetic and chemical. Any human being who had these chemical imbalances would act similarly. We don't see diabetes in the mental health bible, yet people with low blood sugar might act nasty or drunk even though they are *not* drunk. Similarly, people who are bipolar might act crazy even though they are *not* crazy. There are excellent medications now for bipolar disorder that prevent mood swings and mania. These medications work for the majority of people with bipolar disorder.

There are two schools of thought on mental illness. One school says that it's significantly different behavior and the other school says that it's the extreme of normalcy. Who of us has not had a "manic moment" when we have done something outside the norm? The tie breaker is whether it makes a person's life unmanageable.

But what if they go crazy? Actually, less than 2 percent of the bipolar population becomes psychotic from bipolar disorder. Nevertheless, we seem to make the rules for the other 98 percent based on that 2 percent.

Ignorance of bipolar disorder is costing us $7 billion a year in healthcare costs, more than $40 billion a year in forensic costs, and the loss of some of the most brilliant and innovative people. Winston Churchill was bipolar. Churchill was a great leader despite his bipolar disorder. There is a long list of people who are bipolar who could think outside the box. They are Mother Nature's brilliant pioneers. If you build a faster train, there is more risk of derailment once in a while. Don't throw the genius babies out with the bathwater.

People who are bipolar and not on medication tend to have mood swings in which their brains are momentarily connected to their tongues. Most of us can stop ourselves from saying things we might *like* to say but don't say because we see the bigger picture. People who are bipolar do not always have that luxury when they are manic. Others take what they say personally. When someone is manic, hasn't slept for three days, and is obviously in a mood, we need to take that into consideration. I get tired of filling out the questionnaire for my patients on the application for Social Security: "Can this person work?" My real answer would be "Yes, if the boss would stop firing him." The bipolar person has a manic moment and tells the boss off, and the boss takes it personally and fires him. With a little bit of education, the boss might be able to see that it's just a mood swing. If it's not a mood swing then bipolar disorder should not be used as an excuse. You would be surprised at how many "closet bipolars" are out there, afraid to admit they're bipolar because they may lose their job, their dignity, and their standing in the community. Practical education of the general public is necessary if we mean it when we say that everyone is created equal. Without realizing it, we are pushing away some of the cream of the crop.

Fred's Note

Kristin told me, early in our relationship, that she had bipolar disorder. I didn't have any knowledge about this chemical imbalance, but I saw that Kristin's treatment seemed similar to the way that a diabetic manages diabetes. Both can require an adjustment in your daily lifestyle. She took lithium to keep her bipolar symptoms under control. Prior to Kristin's going off her medication, bipolar disorder had no real effect on our relationship. She took a risk in disclosing it to me, not knowing how I would react. I truly appreciated her honesty!

Kristin's courage during her two pregnancies is nothing short of amazing—especially during her first pregnancy. Initially, we were both discouraged after our genetic counseling session when we learned about the risks that lithium could have on our unborn baby. Going off lithium was a gamble for Kristin, because she didn't fully know how her mind would react. I know there were times when her mind was racing wildly or when she was feeling depressed. She must have wondered if we had made the right decision to have a family. Her desire to have a healthy baby kept her focused and helped her to overcome these questions in her mind.

Kristin recorded her problems after the birth of our first child: the effects of being off lithium, back spasms, breast infections, and heavy bleeding. We faced these challenges together and managed to overcome them. Again, her endurance and faith were paramount in the nine weeks after Katherine was born.

After everything Kristin went through with our first child, I was surprised when she suggested that we try to have a second child two years later. However, she again displayed confidence and determination to have another healthy baby, and our second daughter Holly was born.

As a newborn, Holly required much more care than Katherine. We called her our "high-maintenance" baby. She was often fussy, did not sleep through the night, and just needed extra attention. I think the stress of having a newborn along with a two-and-a-half-year-old took its toll on Kristin. After one month, we decided it would be best for her to resume lithium. I knew that Kristin wanted to breastfeed longer, but she had to consider her own health. I think she did a wonderful job handling a tough situation for as long as she did.

I have been astonished by Kristin's effort to write this book. You normally think of someone who writes a self-help book as having an advanced degree in a medical field and doing years of research. Kristin has successfully managed two pregnancies while off medication. In addition to the extensive research she has done, she utilized the journals and diaries she kept over many years. Kristin's motive for writing this book is a strong desire to help others who have bipolar disorder and those who don't understand the nature of this chemical imbalance. I believe that she has succeeded in meeting her objectives.

When she first told me she planned to write a book, I encouraged her to pursue her desire but urged her not to let it consume her. Because of her bipolar disorder, even though it is under control, she has a tendency to become so involved in a task that she forgets to make time for some of the other aspects of her life. However, our relationship has not suffered, nor has it interfered with her time spent with our children. It is Kristin's leisure time that has been most affected. She told me many times how much she enjoyed working on this book. She has described it as her labor of love!

There were periods while Kristin was writing the book that I thought if I heard the word *bipolar* one more time, I would become bipolar myself! But my few frustrations pale in comparison to what she has gone through in completing her marathon. Watching her pour herself into this book and handling all the details necessary to get it published is a testament to her commitment to helping people. Kristin's devotion to this project has been nothing short of awe-inspiring to all those around her.

Epilogue

Many of our days have been filled with magic and excitement. Those memories will last forever. Fred and I encountered some tough periods along the way, but they were all temporary. We took one day at a time, remained positive, and sought advice when it was needed.

The first time I read through this book in its final stage, I realized that together, Fred and I had conquered something big. We have our own family now, and I couldn't be more proud. I envisioned myself on top of a mountain, saying, "We did it!" In the beginning, we felt apprehension, excitement, and determination once we decided to have a family, but we put our plan into action and fulfilled it.

That actually sounds simple, but it wasn't. My marriage with Fred became stronger during these challenging times. The work, commitment, and dedication we both displayed drew us even closer together.

Because Fred and I modified our lives for a short time and made necessary sacrifices, we are now blessed with two healthy, wonderful daughters: Katherine Kay and Holly Marie. They are vastly different individuals, as most siblings are.

Katherine enjoys choir, swimming, downhill skiing, running, talking on the phone, and shopping. Holly likes Tae Kwon Do, baseball, hanging out with friends, and playing guitar. Both like to spend time at their grandma and grandpa's beautiful home on Lake Michigan—especially if boating or downhill skiing is involved.

My goal in this book has been to provide a road map for those who share the same dream that Fred and I had: to have a family. If you are bipolar, embrace it. Channel and manage your bipolar gifts, and experience contentment and freedom. Embracing bipolar disorder will help you to live your dreams.

Appendix A

Genetic Counseling

HELGA VALDMANIS TORIELLO, Ph.D.

When you receive genetic counseling, you will hear a number of terms with which you might not be familiar. Please refer to the glossary for an explanation of genetic terms.

Bipolar disorder (BPD) is a relatively common condition that clearly has a genetic component. This is based on family, twin, and adoption studies that indicate that biological family members of those with BPD have a greater chance of themselves developing BPD, and that heritability of the condition is estimated to be 58 to 74 percent (Fallin et al., 2004). The cause of BPD is thought to be caused by both genetic and environmental factors. In addition, there are likely to be different genes involved, with one group of genes responsible for BPD in some families, and a different group of genes responsible for BPD in other families (Fallin et al., 2004). Given this genetic component, individuals who have BPD themselves, or who have a family history of BPD, often seek genetic counseling to determine what their chances are of having a child who will be similarly affected. In addition, women who have BPD and are on one or more medications for the management of their condition are often concerned about the possible risk posed by these medications for a developing fetus. Therefore, genetic counseling is often sought either before planning a pregnancy or after a pregnancy is detected, to obtain more information about potential risks.

Genetic Counseling: Definition and History

The term *genetic counseling* was first coined nearly sixty years ago (Reed, 1949). By the early 1950s, numerous "hereditary disorders" or "hereditary counseling" clinics were established across the United States. In these clinics, physicians with training in genetics saw patients with family histories of genetic disorders and focused on the provision of recurrence risks. However, as the role of genetics professionals expanded to include diagnosis, discussion of testing options, and so forth, the need for these individuals to provide at least some of these services arose.

In response to the continuing need for increasing the number of trained professionals to provide clinical genetic counseling, the field of genetic counseling was born at Sarah Lawrence College, where the first class of trained genetic counselors graduated in 1971 (Baker, Schuette, & Uhlmann, 1998). The National Society of Genetic Counselors (NSCG) was then established in

1975, and it included, as of 2002, 1,020 certified genetic counselors (CGCs). CGCs are full members who are certified by the American Board of Genetic Counseling or the American Board of Medical Genetics to practice genetic counseling and agree to abide by the established code of ethics of the NSGC.

In 1975, the American Society of Human Genetics adopted the following definition of genetic counseling: "Genetic counseling is a communication process which deals with the human problems associated with the occurrence or risk of occurrence of a genetic disorder in a family."

The process involves several steps that will be detailed later in this appendix.

The Goals of Genetics Evaluation and Genetic Counseling

Genetic counseling is an integral part of genetics evaluation, which includes diagnosis; interpretation of genetic (molecular, chromosomal, and biochemical) test results; cause, if known; recurrence risk; prognosis (natural history and course of the condition); and treatment options. It also includes counseling directed toward the patient's clarification of concerns; assessment of family issues; processing of information; development of decision-making and coping strategies; referrals for medical, psychological, and support group follow-up; and general promotion of the client's psychosocial health. There is no single formula that serves as a one-size-fits-all approach; in the hands of experienced genetics professionals, a specific genetics session will vary according to the patient's and family's needs at that time (Baker, Schuette, & Uhlmann, 1998; Kenen & Smith, 1995; Kessler, 1992).

Typically a patient is seen by one or more board-certified genetics professionals, including a medical geneticist, a genetic counselor, and/or a genetic nurse (Baker, Schuette, & Uhlmann, 1998). Since the inception of the practice of genetic counseling, there has been a debate about who is qualified to provide genetic counseling services. This debate continues, spurred in part by the projected continuing increase in referrals for genetic counseling and the dearth of genetic counselors who hold CGC certification (Greendale & Pyeritz, 2001; Guttmacher, Jenkins, & Uhlmann, 2001; Kenen & Smith, 1995; Touchette, Holtzman, Davis, & Feetham, 1997).

The Stages of Genetic Counseling

Genetic counseling is a time-consuming process that involves a number of steps (Tsuang, Faraone, & Tsuang, 2001). The first step is the confirmation of the diagnosis. This generally involves requesting medical records from the treating physicians to determine whether the diagnosis of the condition for which the individual is seeking counseling is indeed correct. For example, symptoms consistent with bipolar disorder can be seen in Wilson's disease, which is a genetic condition that causes the accumulation of copper in various organs (Ferenci, 1998; Keller,

Torta, Lagget, Crasto, & Bergamasco, 1999). The inheritance of Wilson's disease is autosomal recessive, so the chance of an individual with Wilson's disease having a similarly affected child would be approximately 1 in 180 (Figus et al., 1989). The second step is the review of the family history. The general standard is to obtain a three-generation pedigree, and to include first-degree (children, siblings, and parents), second-degree (nieces, nephews, aunts, uncles, half-siblings, and grandparents), and third-degree (cousins, great-grandparents, and siblings' grandchildren) relatives. Information about the mental health of these individuals is crucial to the determination of recurrence risks. In some cases, medical records might have to be requested to verify reported diagnoses.

After these first and second steps have been completed, the third step—the assessment of the recurrence risk—can be done. There are several sources of information on genetic risks that can be consulted. In general, however, an individual with no family history of bipolar disorder has a 1 percent chance of developing it, but the chance of a first-degree relative developing it is 9–14 percent, and that person's chance of developing depression is 14–42 percent (Chang, Steiner, & Ketter, 2003; Joyce et al., 2004).

These risks are modified by factors such as the number of affected family members and the age of onset in family members, with increased numbers of affected family members and earlier age of onset in family members conferring a greater risk (Craddock & Jones, 1999; Pauls, Morton, & Egeland, 1992).

There is also evidence that bipolar disorder is heterogeneous (i.e., it has different causes), and this can also influence risks. For example, different forms of bipolar disorder, such as lithium-responsive versus lithium-nonresponsive, or bipolar disorder associated with rapid cycling versus seasonal affective disorder, are almost certainly caused by different susceptibility genes (Craddock & Jones, 1999; Demidenko, Grof, Alda, Deshauer, & Duffy, 2004).

Finally, discussions of recurrence risk should also include the risks for related conditions. Recent studies have suggested that the chance of the child of a bipolar parent having a psychiatric disorder is approximately 50 percent (Chang et al., 2003; Reichart, Wals, Hillegers, Ormel, Nolen, & Verhulst, 2004). Once the risks are determined, the counselor must convey this information to the consultant and help him or her to integrate this information together with the perceived burdens of the condition.

This is not a straightforward process. Conditions that have a high risk of recurrence but available treatment may be regarded as more "acceptable" than disorders that have a low recurrence risk but no treatment (and thus a debilitating effect on the individual). Therefore, genetic counseling must provide a forum for the consultant to integrate the risk factors with the burden of the condition and patient's values.

The final step is the development of a plan of action. For many conditions, this includes the options of prenatal or presymptomatic testing (i.e., testing before symptoms appear). Currently this is not an option for bipolar disorder, for which causative genes have not yet been identified. However, as genes are identified, molecular testing will be an option for some families, particularly those in which the condition appears to be inherited as an autosomal dominant trait and thus caused by a single gene (Radhakrishna et al., 2001).

How Do We Know That Bipolar Disorder Is Genetic?

There is clear evidence that BPD has a genetic component, based on family, adoption, and twin studies. Family studies suggest that a particular condition is genetic by demonstrating a higher incidence in family members than would be expected by chance. For example, whereas the population frequency of BPD is thought to be approximately 1 percent, the chance of a closely related family member having BPD can be as high as 9 percent, or nine times the frequency found in the general population.

To separate out shared environmental influences, studies also look at the frequency in identical versus fraternal twins and adopted children whose biological parents have BPD (Belmaker, 2004; Craddock & Jones, 1999; Smoller & Finn, 2003). Identical twins are more than twice as likely as fraternal twins to *both* be affected with bipolar disorder (thus indicating genetic influence, since identical twins have all their genes in common, compared to fraternal twins, who have only half their genes in common). Adopted individuals who develop

BPD are almost three times as likely to have a biological parent with BPD than to have an adoptive parent with BPD (Smoller & Finn, 2003).

When Should a Woman with Bipolar Disorder Receive Genetic Counseling?

The ideal time for genetic counseling is preconception; that is, before attempting a pregnancy. However, since almost half of all pregnancies in the general population are unplanned, it is recommended to begin counseling as soon as the pregnancy is diagnosed.

Teratology is the name given to the study of abnormal embryonic or fetal development. A *teratogen* is any substance that causes damage to the developing embryo or fetus, ranging from loss of the embryo to behavioral and/or cognitive problems in the exposed child. To determine if a particular substance is a teratogen, several variables must be taken into account. First is the timing of the exposure. Most development of organs occurs between the second and ninth weeks after conception (before many women even know they're pregnant). Before that time, there is an all-or-none phenomenon—that is, either the embryo is miscarried or no effect from the teratogen occurs. After that time, almost all development is completed, so exposure to a teratogen will not cause malformations (birth defects).

Second is dosage and frequency of exposure. For many substances, a higher dose poses a greater risk. In addition, a single exposure is considered less risky than chronic exposure. Third is the concept of fetal susceptibility. It is known that not every fetus that is exposed to a potentially teratogenic substance will be affected. Similarly, even within the same family, one exposed child could have no ill effects while another has multiple birth defects and mental retardation. It is likely that certain genes confer increased susceptibility or relative resistance to a potential teratogen's effects.

Last is the quality of the data by which the assessments are made. At least half of the available data on a particular substance comes from animal studies (Conover, 1994). The problem with such studies is that animals are usually exposed to dosages much higher than those used in humans, and animals often have different susceptibilities to some of these substances. In many other cases, the only human data consist of single case reports (e.g., a birth defect in a child prenatally exposed to a new type of medication).

Although these cases can be helpful in leading to more detailed studies of a group of exposed children, in themselves they are not sufficient to suggest that a substance is teratogenic. That being said, there does appear to be fairly decent information on many of the medications used to treat BPD. Table A-1 gives a summary of what was known as of December 2006. Another good source of information on medications and their effect on pregnancy is available at www.otispregnancy.org.

It should be stressed that the time to discuss medication regimens and pregnancy should be before conception. However, when a woman with BPD discovers that she is pregnant, she should not change or discontinue her medications until she discusses it with her primary care physician. It is also important that she immediately consult with her ob-gyn.

Table A-1. BPD Medications and Risks to the Fetus for Anomalies

Medication	Condition (risk)	Strength of data	References
Lithium	Cardiac defects (1%–4%), Ebstein anomaly (0.1%–0.2%). Neonatal hypothyroidism, diabetes insipidus, macrosomia (rare). Overall risk of anomalies, 4%–12%.	Fair to good. Several hundred pregnancies have been studied.	Dodd & Berk (2004); Ernst & Goldberg (2002); Iqbal et al. (2001); TERIS website; Viguera et al. (2002); Yonkers et al. (2004); Grover et al. (2006)
Depakote (valproic acid)	Spina bifida (1%–5%), limb defects (0.5%), developmental delay/MR (30%). Fetal valproate syndrome (can be as high as 25%). Risks seem to be associated with dosages of 1,000 mg/day or more.	Fair to good	Dodd & Berk (2004); Ernst & Goldberg (2002); Gagliardi & Krishnan (2003); Iqbal et al. (2001); Jager-Roman et al. (1986); Shepard et al. (2002); Teratogenic Information Systems (TERIS) website

Table A-1 (continued)

Medication	Condition (risk)	Strength of data	References
Tegretol (carbamazepine)	Spina bifida (1%–2%); fetal carbamazepine syndrome (10%–20%); Birth defects in general (5%–6%)	Fair to good	Dodd & Berk (2004); Ernst & Goldberg (2002); Gagliardi & Krishnan (2003); Iqbal et al. (2001); TERIS website; Yonkers et al. (2004)
Thorazine	Insignificant, if any, increased risk for malformations	Fair to good	TERIS website; Grover et al. (2006)
Haldol (haloperidol)	Insignificant, if any, increased risk for malformations	Fair	TERIS website
Mellaril (thioridazine)	Unknown, but risk considered low	Limited	TERIS website; Reprotox website
Lamictal (lamotrigine)	Small, if any, increased risk for major malformations (5% or less)	Fair	Reprotox website; Tennis et al. (2002); TERIS website; Grover et al. (2006)
Topamax (topiramate)	Unknown	Limited	Ernst & Goldberg (2002); Reprotox website; TERIS website; Grover et al. (2006)
Neurontin (gabapentin)	Unknown, but may be as high as 6% for birth defects	Limited	Ernst & Goldberg (2002); TERIS website

Table A-1 (continued)

Medication	Condition (risk)	Strength of data	References
Gabitril (tiagabine)	Unknown	Limited	TERIS website
Trileptal (oxcarbazepine)	Could be similar to carbamazepine	Limited	Reprotox website
Abilify (aripiprazole)	Unknown	None	TERIS website; Reprotox website
Zyprexa (olanzapine)	Unknown, but unlikely to be above 5%	Limited	Ernst & Goldberg (2002); TERIS website; Grover et al. (2006)
Geodon (ziprasidone)	Unknown	Limited	Ernst & Goldberg (2002); TERIS website
Seroquel (quetiapine)	Unknown	Limited (one case reported; normal outcome)	Ernst & Goldberg (2002); Reprotox website; Grover et al. (2006)
Clozaril (clozapine)	Some risk cannot be excluded.	Limited (based on case reports of infants with anomalies)	Ernst & Goldberg (2002); TERIS website; Grover et al. (2006)

Appendix B

Becoming Pregnant

JUDITH HIEMENGA, M.D.

W hen there is an existing family history of bipolar disorder, children are also at risk. This is a good time to see a genetic counselor. Any of us can have additional health risks, such as heart disease, osteoporosis, or breast cancer. The incidence of birth defects in the general population is 3–5 percent. Those defects can range from very minor to severe and life threatening. Considering this, bipolar disorder is just another manageable illness and usually doesn't prevent a person from living life to the fullest.

Long-term pre-pregnancy planning is especially important for those who are bipolar. Since you are unique, adapt pre-pregnancy suggestions from your physician to fit your situation and circumstances. As you read further, you'll see that I'm describing a best-case scenario in a near-perfect world. Do you have medical insurance to cover prenatal care, delivery, and postpartum expenses? There are other financial considerations for the bipolar woman. You might need to take extra time off work during and after pregnancy. Your partner might need time off work to help with your new baby.

It's best if you're healthy prior to pregnancy. See your primary care physician for a routine physical exam. Schedule an appointment with your ob-gyn for a preconception checkup. Get into the routine of eating a balanced diet, getting adequate sleep, and exercising regularly. Start taking prenatal vitamin supplements (including folic acid). A psychiatric consultation and some psychological counseling can help to increase your emotional stability. Continued counseling might be helpful during the hormonal roller coaster of pregnancy. If possible, you should be stabilized off medication prior to conception.

Consider the ideal time of year for pregnancy, especially if your prior bipolar symptom flare-ups have been seasonal. The short, dark days of winter could impact your emotional risks with increased depressive symptoms associated with seasonal affective disorder. Conception just prior to or during shorter winter days might be ideal, so that the remaining six to eight months of pregnancy fall during the longer, brighter days of spring and summer. With a spring or summer delivery, most postpartum recovery occurs prior to the gloomy months of November and December. This will also allow more flexibility in getting out of the house with your baby.

Confinement for long periods of time at home with limited social interaction is difficult for anyone, but especially for bipolar women. Tumultuous postpartum hormonal changes increase the risk of postpartum depression. It may be recommended by your psychiatrist that you restart bipolar disorder medication if you've chosen not to breastfeed.

Watching for significant psychiatric flare-ups of depression or mania for one or two cycles before conception can be helpful in predicting how you will tolerate medication changes. During the same two months off all psychiatric medications, oral contraceptives can be discontinued. Contraceptive foam and condoms, contraceptive gel and condoms, or a diaphragm with contraceptive gel should be substituted for birth control pills before conceiving. This will establish your body's own menstrual cycle rather than the cycle regulated by birth control pills.

Normal hormonal changes cause many women to experience premenstrual syndrome (PMS), with symptoms such as food cravings (especially sweets), moodiness, irritability, anger, anxiety, disturbed sleep patterns, and fatigue. Physical symptoms such as bloating, constipation, fluid retention, and breast pain or tenderness are common. Make the following positive changes:

- Avoid caffeine and alcohol.
- Eat more protein, complex carbohydrates, and fiber. Increase nutrients such as calcium (1,200 mg) daily and vitamin B^6 (25 mg) twice daily.
- Exercise throughout the day.
- Get plenty of sleep.

• Keep a journal to track symptoms suggestive of a bipolar episode and also the dates of your periods.

The menstrual cycle usually averages twenty-eight days. It begins the first day of a woman's period, which lasts five to seven days. Ovulation usually occurs about day 14. After ovulation the egg is alive from twelve to twenty-four hours. During that twelve hours, many women will experience the slight aching or pelvic discomfort called *mittelschmerz* (a German term meaning "mid-pain"). After intercourse, sperm survive up to forty-eight hours in the cervical mucus, uterine fluid, and fallopian tubes. Ejaculated sperm move on their own and by uterine contractions and specialized cells in the fallopian tubes that transport them. The sperm and egg meet within minutes rather than hours.

Most fertile couples will achieve pregnancy within a year; 80 percent of these will be pregnant in six months. When you have regular menstrual cycles, planning and attempting conception is easier. Since the menstrual cycle is variable, timing can be both difficult and frustrating. Predicting ovulation can be made easier by keeping a calendar of your menstrual cycle. Purchase a basal digital thermometer at a pharmacy. Included are specific instructions and a chart explaining temperature variations and why they occur. Ovulation predictor kits can be helpful for some couples.

Many techniques can be used to optimize the chances of conception. With each menstrual cycle that results in ovulation, perfect timing for intercourse can still result in only a 25 percent chance of conception. Consider these additional recommendations, if applicable. Your genetics clinic consultation will address maternal age if you are over thirty-five. If you need to continue your bipolar medications during pregnancy, the drugs with the lowest risk should be used, especially in the first three months.

With infrequent or irregular cycles, you might need to see an infertility specialist or a reproductive endocrinologist. Men should consider an evaluation of their sperm count and motility. A woman over age thirty-five should be evaluated to see if her hormones suggest a premenopausal decrease in fertility.

Intercourse every forty-eight hours from day 10 to day 17 will optimize conception for most couples. If your cycle varies in length, ovulation time will vary. However, the time from ovulation to the start of your period tends to be consistent at fourteen days. When looking at previous cycles you've charted on your calendar, you can only guess when ovulation will occur as you count *forward.* You can predict, fairly accurately, when you've ovulated before the start of your period. By having intercourse at least every forty-eight hours from four to five days before ovulation until three to four days after ovulation, the chances of conceiving improve, even if your cycle is slightly irregular.

Immediately before ovulation, high estrogen levels stimulate secretion of a large amount of thin clear watery mucus that is hospitable to sperm transit. After ovulation, high progesterone levels stimulate secretion of a scant, thick, white mucus that is less hospitable to sperm. Check your own vaginal secretions and record the information on your calendar.

If conception has occurred on day 14, the fertilized egg will be transported through the fallopian tube to the uterine cavity over a one-week period. At approximately day 21, or seven days after ovulation and conception, the fertilized egg implants in the uterine wall. Two to three days after implantation, human chorionic gonadotropin (HCG) (a hormone produced by the placenta in pregnancy) is detectable in the bloodstream. By day 28, a pregnancy test could have been positive for three to five days if conception has taken place. If conception hasn't occurred, you have a period, and a new cycle starts.

If your menstrual cycle is extremely irregular, especially if it is longer than forty days, fertility drugs might be necessary. Without intervention, you have fewer chances in a year to conceive, which might lengthen the time you have to be off your bipolar medication. Infrequent ovulation and menstruation require a special evaluation of the risks and benefits of fertility drugs. With prompt, appropriate intervention, couples usually conceive as planned and have less chance of a high-risk pregnancy.

Appendix C

Postpartum Disorders

INGRID EERDMANS, M.D.

The postpartum period is generally defined as the time from birth to one year thereafter. It is a time of such dramatic change and adjustment biologically, psychologically, and socially that it is difficult to fully appreciate it until you're immersed in it. So much time is spent trying to juggle the simplest routine tasks, like showering or sleeping, around the baby's needs that there is precious little time left to attend to one's own emotional and mental status. However, this cannot be neglected, because the postpartum period has many associated disorders. These conditions can have serious consequences for the entire family and must be quickly identified and treated.

There are three degrees of postpartum disorder: blues, depression, and psychosis.

Postpartum Blues

Postpartum blues, or "baby blues," affect 50–80 percent of women who give birth, making it the most common postpartum disorder. The symptoms generally begin three to five days after birth, although they may occur as early as the first day. They peak in five to ten days. The syndrome is usually resolved by two weeks after delivery. Postpartum blues seem to occur in most cultures, although studies of African and Asian women indicate that they express their depressive symptoms in physical terms, like headaches and other pains, rather than in psychological terms, as American women seem to do. Crying is the primary symptom for American women. Additional complaints in American women include loneliness, sensitivity to rejection, irritability, anxiety, confusion, indecision, insomnia, exhaustion, fear, and loss of sexual interest.

No definitive purpose or cause for the blues has been substantiated, but many theories have been proposed. One evolutionary hypothesis holds that the blues are a positive trait that increases a woman's vigilance after childbirth and improves her infant's chance of survival. The blues can also provide a release function that allows a woman to relieve herself of the intense anxiety surrounding childbirth.

Biological theories have focused on changing levels of hormones or, perhaps more important, their rapid rate of change. However, specific levels of estrogen, progesterone, prolactin, thyroid, and cortisol do not always correlate well with symptoms, and external hormone manipulations, especially with supplements, has not generally been an effective treatment. The amino acid tryptophan has decreased circulatory levels during pregnancy, but it normally increases in the first five days after birth. One study found lower than normal levels of circulating tryptophan in depressed postpartum women. However, this is probably just a marker for some unknown causative factor, because supplementation with tryptophan doesn't reduce the blues.

Some hold that the blues are a stress reaction, because women who have had surgery experience a similar mood postoperatively. It is interesting to note that the rate of postpartum blues is the same after both vaginal and cesarean deliveries. It could be that the actual beginning of the blues is masked or delayed by relief and excitement after delivery, which results in a brief postpartum euphoria.

The postpartum blues usually resolve spontaneously. The condition is made more tolerable with good supportive care, primarily involving steps to minimize fatigue and isolation. Emotional support can come from a spouse or partner, extended family members, other mothers, and your nurse, midwife, or physician. Prevention of fatigue is facilitated by specific help with housework, sleeping when the baby sleeps, an occasional change of scene, exercise and healthy diet, delaying big decisions, and allowing for imperfection. Acknowledge that your new life is not the same while recognizing that it's still a good life and focusing on its positive aspects.

Postpartum Depression

Postpartum depression (PPD) occurs in 10–20 percent of women after delivery. Twenty percent of women with baby blues go on to develop PPD. Women who have suffered a previous depression anytime in their lives have a 30 percent greater chance of developing PPD. Women who have had a previous bout of PPD have a 50–80 percent chance of having PPD after a subsequent pregnancy. The incidence of PPD is 30 percent for women living in poverty. There are no racial or ethnic differences in overall prevalence, but African-American and Hispanic women report symptoms earlier than Caucasian women. It is important to recognize that 4 percent of postpartum fathers develop PPD. This condition occurs in adoptive parents as well.

Although onset most commonly occurs in the fourth week after delivery, it can develop anytime between birth and the first year thereafter. There is controversy time frame, just as there is about most aspects of postpartum disorder. The *Diagnostic and Statistical Manual* (DSM-IV), the American Psychiatric Association's manual for diagnosing and coding psychiatric disorders, categorizes PPD as a major depressive disorder that occurs in the postpartum period. However, the manual limits the postpartum period to the first four months after delivery. The International Coding System (a widely accepted system for defining and coding psychiatric disorders, similar to the DSM-IV) defines postpartum as the first six months after delivery. However, most researchers define the postpartum period as the first year after delivery.

Symptoms of PPD include many of the same symptoms of the blues, but they are more intense, unremitting, and disabling. There can also be a progressive worsening of symptoms: from feeling blue to anxiety and panic attacks to worthlessness to suicidal thoughts. These mothers can develop unbidden fantasies about hurting their child that are frightening and repulsive to them. They might begin avoiding their baby to avoid triggering these horrifying thoughts.

Additional symptoms include the following: sad or depressed mood, irritability, indecision, fatigue, trouble sleeping (even if given the opportunity to do so), anxiety, fear, crying, anhedonia (loss of interest in usually pleasurable activities), low libido, feelings of worthlessness, inability to cope, poor self-care, feeling like a bad mother, feelings of guilt and shame, a desire to isolate oneself from others, and poor concentration. Associated physical complaints may include dry skin, fluid retention, constipation, headaches, and panic symptoms, such as chest pain, dizziness, limb numbness and tingling, flushing, shortness of breath, and nausea. Women with a history of substance abuse, including alcohol and nicotine, are at risk of increasing their use of the substance if they are depressed during pregnancy or the postpartum period.

Risk factors for postpartum depression are many and varied. Those with the strongest correlation to PPD are a personal past history of depression or anxiety disorder, marital discord, poor social supports, and stressful negative life events. Negative events include the death of a close relative or friend, an accident or ill health in a close family member, an undesired move, job loss, or a high-risk or unwanted pregnancy. Additional risks include a history of having had poor mothering; a history of victimization, including childhood abuse or neglect; a tendency to self-blame; having an overly high expectation of oneself; a history of significant PMS; a history of an eating disorder; a difficult infant; short maternity leave; a history of bipolar disorder; a family history of depression or anxiety; and a history of severe baby blues or hypomania after delivery. Age is also a risk factor; studies of adolescents reveal that they have high rates of PPD.

Causation theories for postpartum depression that center on rapidly fluctuating hormonal levels were mentioned previously, in the discussion of postpartum blues. These fluctuations may be coupled with a sluggish response from the pituitary gland. Another theory looks at a desynchronization of normal circadian ("body clock" rhythms) as a factor in PPD. This system normally involves melatonin, cortisol, thyroid-stimulating hormone, and prolactin, which may be altered in the birth process. Treatments aimed at this system—including bright light therapy (>2500 LUX) or wake therapy (sleep deprivation) at specific times of the day—have demonstrated some preliminary benefits. In addition, PPD is associated with thyrotoxicosis in 5–9 percent of cases and with hypothyroidism in 10–15 percent of women with PPD.

Treatment for postpartum depression is imperative. Unfortunately, 50–80 percent of insomnia with PPD remains undetected and untreated. This is due in part to health providers, partners, and the mothers themselves failing to recognize the symptoms, and also in part to the mothers' reluctance to disclose them. Given a lack of education about these disorders, some women think that they must be the only ones to have ever experienced this level of depression after delivery. They are ashamed to admit that they are so unhappy at a time at which they expected to be joyful. These mothers might worry that if anyone knew about their panic attacks, frightening fantasies, and depression, they would be hospitalized and lose custody of their baby. They may feel beyond hope for recovery.

Real consequences occur when postpartum depression goes untreated; the symptoms can last three to twelve months. In fact, 10 percent of women with untreated PPD still have symptoms one year after delivery. This results in difficulty in the bonding process; mothers who are depressed and simply going through the motions do not look and smile at their baby as much, and their babies begin to withdraw. These babies can grow up to see the world as a sad place. Infants exposed to a depressed mother for more than two months have less weight gain, and they are more likely to be depressed, anxious, or aggressive themselves. They are more likely to have lower cognitive skills and experience long-term delays in social, emotional, and speech development.

Children of depressed parents are at higher risk for early-onset major depressive disorders, alcohol abuse, and medical problems. Maternal PPD places significant stress on a marriage and tremendous additional unanticipated burdens on the father. Finally, the longer the depression goes untreated, the more treatment-resistant it becomes.

Treatment is multifaceted. Educational information should be offered at an early prenatal office visit and in the initial postpartum period. Recognizing the importance of this, New Jersey recently passed a law requiring doctors to educate expectant mothers and their families about postpartum depression and to screen new mothers for this condition. Simple screening questionnaires should be administered during pregnancy, at postpartum visits, and ideally at well-child visits to the pediatrician or family physician in the first year.

Supportive measures, like those mentioned in the treatment of postpartum blues, are also essential here. In addition, the depressed mother should be encouraged to set small achievable goals and to give herself credit for the work she is doing. She should be allowed to acknowledge that caring for an infant is hard work. Her diet should include plenty of vegetables, fruits, and water. Junk food, alcohol, caffeine, and sugary drinks should be avoided.

It is especially important for the husband not to expect himself to be his wife's sole source of support. His most important roles are to monitor symptoms, advocate for treatment, ensure that the prescribed treatment is followed, and validate her feelings of depression. He needs to address his own feelings as well.

In mild cases of postpartum depression, therapy alone can significantly improve the symptoms. A postpartum support group or therapists familiar with treating PPD are most effective. If a woman has experienced PPD in prior pregnancies, beginning therapy during a subsequent pregnancy can delay the need for medication, should PPD recur. Joint sessions with the spouse are often helpful in identifying issues and copying strategies.

Medication treatment is often necessary for postpartum depression. Selective serotonin reuptake inhibitors (SSRIs) are usually the medication of choice; these include Prozac, Paxil, Zoloft, Celexa, Lexapro, Effexor, and Luvox. Zoloft is most frequently used, especially if the woman is breastfeeding, because it is virtually undetectable in breast milk unless the mother is taking more than 100 mg a day. Because women who have recently given birth are often sensitive to medication side effects, treatment should begin at 25 mg a day, which is half the usually recommended starting dose. Benzodiazepine, such as Ativan, for the treatment of accompanying anxiety, should be avoided. These are highly excreted in breast milk and can cause slowed breathing in the baby. Medication should improve depressive symptoms gradually over four to eight weeks and should be continued for six months to prevent relapse. Women who have experienced PPD with prior pregnancies should consider starting an antidepressant in the last trimester or immediately after delivery as a preventative measure.

Medication issues aside, breastfeeding should be discussed thoroughly with a mother with postpartum disorder. Even if she is stressed by it, she might be very reluctant to discontinue it because in her depressed, worthless-feeling, negative state, she sees breastfeeding as the only way to still connect with her child and provide good care. On the other hand, it will be a relief for her to be presented with options and available supports in a nonjudgmental fashion.

Postpartum Psychosis

Postpartum psychosis (PPP) is a medical emergency that occurs in 1–4 of every 1,000 postpartum women. Though rare, this is the condition that makes for horrifying national headlines: There is a risk of infanticide in 4 percent of these cases. There is also a significant risk of maternal suicide. Prompt recognition and treatment of this disorder are paramount.

Symptoms of PPP begin three to fourteen days after delivery 75 percent of the time. Another 10 percent of cases will have occurred by one month after delivery. Early symptoms can mimic postpartum blues or PPD, with sleep disturbance, depression, hypomania, or fatigue. Rapidly, the symptoms of agitation, hyperactivity, insomnia, confusion, hallucinations, delusions, volatile mood shifts, bizarre behavior, and panic develop.

Postpartum psychosis has a strong genetic component. There is controversy over whether it is a distinct entity or a bipolar episode. If the latter, is the bipolar episode genetically prompted by childbirth, simply occurring as a response to stress, or coincidentally occurring after delivery? Whatever the case, if a woman is affected with bipolar disorder and has a family history of a relative who had PPP, she has a 75 percent chance of incurring PPP herself. If she is affected with bipolar but has no family history of PPP, her chance of PPP falls to 30 percent. A large population study in 1987 found that women with bipolar disorder were hospitalized more often for PPP than were women who had a history of schizophrenia or depression. The identified risk factors included being unmarried, having a first baby, undergoing a cesarean delivery, and infant death.

Treatment of postpartum psychosis begins with hospitalization. Even with the use of medication, hospitalization can be lengthy. Therefore, electroconvulsive therapy (ECT), which often results in more rapid symptom remission, can be useful, because there's less time lost for the mother-infant bonding process. In some cases, ECT and medication will be prescribed. ECT is a safe, rapidly effective, widely recognized treatment for a medical emergency.

A Note on Posttraumatic Stress Disorder

Other disorders can arise after delivery due to the rigors of childbirth, the stress of parenting, or simply coincidentally. *Postpartum adjustment disorder,* or stress syndrome; *postpartum obsessive compulsive disorder,* and *postpartum panic disorder* are all identified as distinct disorders in some postpartum literature, but their manifestations lie within the symptom spectrum of PPD. Therefore, they could represent variations of PPD or be coincidentally arising disorders. Preexisting conditions can also be exacerbated by pregnancy, childbirth, and postpartum stressors.

That said, posttraumatic stress disorder (PTSD) after childbirth deserves special mention. It occurs in 1.5–6 percent of postpartum women as a result of birth trauma, an event that occurs during the process of labor and delivery, and involves actual or threatened serious injury or death of the mother or her infant. The risk of PTSD increases if the birthing woman experiences a lack of support from the delivery staff or her partner, especially while requiring a high degree of obstetrical intervention. This can include forceps delivery, emergency C-section, incomplete epidural, or undesired episiotomy. The risk also increases with long, painful labor, a perceived lack of information or options, and differences between the woman's expectations and the actual event. She experiences intense fear, helplessness, loss of control, and even horror. Untreated, the symptoms can persist for life. Treatment consists of processing the events with one of the medical staff present to gather information and correct misperceptions; psychotherapy; and possibly medication, usually an SSRI.

In conclusion, postpartum disorders occur frequently and can have significant consequences. Routine education and screening are essential for early detection of symptoms and subsequent treatment. Like other mental illness, postpartum disorders must be destigmatized in order to minimize their negative effects.

Glossary of Genetic Terms

Allele: One of the forms of a particular gene.

Anticipation: The phenomenon in which a condition appears to develop at an earlier age in the next generation.

Autosomal: One of the numbered chromosomes (as opposed to the sex chromosomes). Males and females are equally affected by autosomal conditions.

Autosomal dominant: A trait that causes a condition to be inherited by a change in one of the alleles. Autosomal dominant traits are generally passed from parent to child, with each child having a 50 percent chance of inheriting the condition from the affected parent.

Autosomal recessive: A trait that causes a condition to be inherited by a change in both alleles. Autosomal recessive traits generally occur in siblings but not parents. The recurrence risk after the birth of an affected child is 25 percent. An individual who has one allele for an autosomal recessive trait is said to be a carrier for that trait.

Chromosome: A structure composed of genes. Human individuals have 23 pairs of chromosomes, 22 of which are the autosomes (numbered 1–22) and 1 of which is the sex chromosome (XX in a female, XY in a male).

Conception: The union of sperm and ovum (egg), the male and female sex cells, in the human body that leads to the development of a new life.

DNA (deoxyribonucleic acid): The double-helix structure of which genes are composed. The components of DNA are nucleic acids, sugars, and phosphates.

Endocrine glands: Any of the ductless glands, such as the adrenals, the thyroid, the pituitary, the ovaries, or the testes, whose secretions pass directly into the bloodstream. The secretions they produce are called hormones.

Estrogen: The primary female sex hormone. A women's estrogen is mainly produced in her ovaries. When the ovaries stop working at menopause, a woman's body will contain very little natural estrogen.

Expressivity: The degree to which a particular trait manifests itself. If a condition has variable expressivity, it can occur in a mild form in one individual and in a severe form in another individual, often within the same family.

Fertilization: The union of the male sperm and female egg (ovum).

Follicle-stimulating hormone (FSH): A hormone released from the pituitary gland in women that is responsible for the development of the egg-containing follicles of the ovaries.

Gene: The basic unit of heredity that codes for a particular product, usually a protein or an enzyme.

Gene mapping: The process of locating on which chromosome a particular gene is located.

Heritability: The proportion of a trait or characteristic that is caused by genetic factors. A trait with 70 percent heritability means that 70 percent of its cause is genetic factors.

Human chorionic gonadotropin (HCG): A hormone produced by the placenta in pregnancy that is necessary for the maintenance of pregnancy. HCG is often given by injection to make the ovary release its egg at the appropriate time in the monthly cycle.

Infertility: A condition in which a supposedly fertile couple does not achieve pregnancy after twelve to eighteen months of regular, normal intercourse.

Mittelshmerz: "Mid-pain." Abdominal discomfort at the time of ovulation.

Multifactorial: A condition that is caused by one or more genes interacting with other genes, environmental factors, or both.

Ovulation: The process in which the egg (ovum) is released from the ovary. In sexually mature females, ovulation usually occurs every twenty-eight days, halfway between the menstrual periods. Ovulation usually starts a fourteen-day chain of events that ends with a menstrual period if pregnancy does not occur.

Penetrance: The state in which an individual with a gene for a particular condition exhibits any manifestations of that condition. Therefore, if a condition has reduced penetrance, not every individual with the causative gene will show the effects of having that gene.

Premenstrual syndrome (PMS): A term applied to the symptoms a woman may experience prior to her menstrual period. They can begin at ovulation and last until the period begins, approximately fourteen days. The symptoms include cramps, backache, tension, depression, irritability, mood swings, swelling, and breast tenderness.

Progesterone: A female hormone produced by the ovaries after ovulation.

X-linked: A condition in which the causative gene is on the X chromosome. In this case, mothers pass the condition to sons, and fathers pass the condition to daughters. Affected men never pass the condition to their sons. Daughters are carriers of one abnormal gene or are "heterozygous." If the gene is dominant, then the daughter is affected; if it is recessive, then the daughter is not affected.

References and Resources

Books and Journal Articles

Abreu, A. (2005). Pharmacologic and hormonal treatments for postpartum depression. *Psychiatric Annals, 35* (7), 568–576.

Baker, D.L., Schuette, J.L., & Uhlmann, W.R. (1998). *A guide to genetic counseling.* New York: Wiley-Liss.

Beck, C. (2004). Birth trauma in the eye of the beholder. *Nursing Research, 53* (1), 28–35.

Belmaker, R.H. (2004). Medical progress: Bipolar disorder. *New England Journal of Medicine, 351,* 476–486.

Beyond the baby blues. (2002). *Parade, 10* (2), 10–12.

Born, L. (2004). Challenges in identifying and diagnosing postpartum disorders. *Primary Psychiatry, 11* (3), 29–36.

Boyer, D.B. (1990). Postpartum depression. *Clinical Issues in Perinatal and Women's Health Nursing, 1* (3), entire issue.

Carter, J. (2006). *Bipolar: The elements of bipolar disorder.* Wyomissing, Pennsylvania: Unicorn Press.

Chang, K., Steiner, H., & Ketter, T. (2003). Studies of offspring of parents with bipolar disorder. *American Journal of Medical Genetics, 123,* 26–35.

Conover, E. (1994). Hazardous exposures during pregnancy. *Journal of Obstetric, Gynecological, and Neonatal Nursing, 23,* 524–532.

Craddock, N., & Jones, I. (1999). Genetics of bipolar disorder. *Journal of Medical Genetics, 36,* 585–594.

Curtis, G., & Schuler, J. (2002). *Your pregnancy journal week by week.* Cambridge, Massachusetts: Perseus.

Demidenko, N., Grof, P., Alda, M., Deshauer, D., & Duffy, A. (2004). MMPI as a measure of sub-threshold and residual psychopathology among the offspring of lithium responsive and non-responsive bipolar parents. *Bipolar Disorders, 6,* 323–328.

Dodd, S., & Berk, M. (2004). The pharmacology of bipolar disorder during pregnancy and breastfeeding. *Expert Opinions on Drug Safety, 3,* 221–229.

Ernst, C.L., & Goldberg, J.F. (2002). The reproductive safety profile of mood stabilizers, atypical antipsychotics, and broad-spectrum psychotropics. *Journal of Clinical Psychiatry, 63* (4), 42–55.

Fallin, M.D., Lasseter, V.K., Wolyniec, P.S., McGrath, J.A., Nestadt, G., Valle, D., Liang, K.Y., & Pulver, A.E. (2004). Genomewide linkage scan for bipolar-disorder susceptibility loci among Ashkenazi Jewish families. *American Journal of Human Genetics, 75,* 204–219.

Fast, Julie A. (2007). The health cards treatment system for bipolar disorder. Self-published.

Ferenci, P. (1998). Wilson's disease. *Clinical Liver Disorders, 2,* 31–49.

Figus, A., Lampis, R., Devoto, M., Ristaldi, M.S., Ideo, A., de Virgilis, S., Nurchi, A.M., Corrias, A., Corda, R., & Lai, M.E. (1989). Carrier detection and early diagnosis of Wilson's disease by restriction fragment length polymorphism analysis. *Journal of Medical Genetics, 26,* 78–82.

Fink, C., & Kraynak, J. (2005). *Bipolar disorder for dummies.* Hoboken, New Jersey: Wiley Publishing.

Flodin, K. (1994). Why new moms get the blues. *Parents, 5,* 71–74.

Flynn H. (2005). Epidemiology and phenomenology of postpartum mood disorders. *Psychiatric Annals, 35* (7), 544–551.

Gagliardi, J.P., & Krishnan, K.R.R. (2003). Evidence-based mental health use of anticonvulsants during pregnancy. *Psychopharmacology Bulletin, 37,* 59–66.

Glover, V. (2004). The biology and pathophysiology of peripartum psychiatric disorders. *Primary Psychiatry, 11* (3), 37–41.

Greendale, K., & Pyeritz, R.E. (2001). Empowering primary care health professionals in medical genetics: How soon? How fast? How far? *American Journal of Medical Genetics, 106,* 223–232.

Grover, S., Avasthi, A., Sharma, Y. (2006). Psychotropics in Pregnancy: Weighing the risks. *Indian Journal of Medical Research, 123,* 497–512.

Gruen, D. (1988). *The new parent: A spectrum of postpartum adjustment.* Mount Sinai Hospital, Toronto: Pennypress.

Guttmacher, A.E., Jenkins, J., & Uhlmann, W.R. (2001). Genomic medicine: Who will practice it? A call to open arms. *American Journal of Medical Genetics, 106,* 216–222.

Hall, L.L., & Renneisen, T. (2004). Managing pregnancy and bipolar disorder. *NAMI Advocate,* Spring/Summer, *1–3.*

Handford, P. (1985). Postpartum depression: What is it, what helps? *Canadian Nurse, 1,* 30–33.

Hodge, A.M. (1997). Postpartum depression: Is it avoidable? *Newsletter of the Council of Childbirth Educators, 3.*

Howell, E.A. (2005). Racial and ethnic difference in factors associated with early postpartum depressive symptoms. *Obstetrics and Gynecology, 105,* 1442–1450.

Iqbal, M.M., Gundlapalli, S.P., Ryan, W.G., Ryals, T., & Passman, T.E. (2001). Effects of antimanic mood-stabilizing drugs on fetuses, neonates, and nursing infants. *Southern Medical Journal, 94,* 304–322.

Jager-Roman, E., Deichl, A., Jakob, S., Hartmann, A.M., Koch, S., Rating, D., Steldinger, R., Nau, H., & Helge, H. (1986). Fetal growth, major malformations, and minor anomalies in infants born to women receiving valproic acid. *Journal of Pediatrics, 108,* 997–1004.

Jones, L. C. (1990). Postpartum emotional disorders. *International Childbirth Education Association (ICEA) Review, 14* (4), 1–8.

Joyce, P.R., Doughty, C.J., Wells, J.E., Walsh, A.E., Admiraal, A., Lill, M., & Olds, R.J. (2004). Affective disorders in the first-degree relatives of bipolar probands: Results from the South Island Bipolar Study. *Comprehensive Psychiatry, 45,* 168–174.

Keller, R., Torta, R., Lagget, M., Crasto, S., & Bergamasco, B. (1999). Psychiatric symptoms as late onset of Wilson's disease: Neuroradiological findings, clinical features and treatment. *Italian Journal of Neurological Science, 20,* 49–54.

Kenen, R.H., & Smith, A.C.M. (1995). Genetic counseling for the next 25 years: Models for the future. *Journal of Genetic Counseling, 4,* 115–124.

Kessler, S. (1992). Psychological aspects of genetic counseling: VII. Thoughts on directiveness. *Journal of Genetic Counseling, 1,* 9–17.

Klinker, D. Postpartum dads. www.postpartumdads.org 2004; 4.

McIlhaney, J. S., & Nethery, S. (1998). *1001 Health-care questions women ask.* Grand Rapids, Michigan: Baker Books.

Melnik, M., Saunders, R., & Saunders, D. (1989). *Managing back pain.* Edina, Minnesota: Educational Opportunities.

Miklowitz, D.J. (2002). *The bipolar disorder survival guide: What you and your family need to know.* New York: Guilford Press.

Murkoff, H., Eisenberg, A., & Hathaway, S. (2002). *What to expect when you're expecting.* New York: Workman.

Murkoff, H. & Mazel, S. (2007). *The what to expect pregnancy journal & organizer.* New York: Workman.

O'Hara, M. (2004). Can postpartum depression be predicted? *Primary Psychiatry, 11* (3), 42–47.

Parry, B. (2004). Treatment of postpartum depression. *Primary Psychiatry, 11* (3), 48–51.

Pauls, D.L., Morton, L.A., & Egeland, J.A. (1992). Risks of affective illness among first-degree relatives of bipolar I old-order Amish probands. *Archives of General Psychiatry, 49,* 703–708.

Radhakrishna, U., Senol, S., Herken, H., Gucuyener, K., Gehrig, C., Blouin, J.L., Akarsu, N.A., & Antonarakis, S.E. (2001). An apparently dominant bipolar affective disorder (BPAD) locus on chromosome 20p11.2-q11.2 in a large Turkish pedigree. *European Journal of Human Genetics, 9,* 39–44.

Reed, S.C. (1949). Counseling in human genetics. *Dight Institute of the University of Minnesota Bulletin, 6,* 7–21.

Reichart, C.G., Wals, M., Hillegers, M.H., Ormel, J., Nolen, W.A., & Verhulst, F.C. (2004). Psychopathology in the adolescent offspring of bipolar parents. *Journal of Affective Disorders, 78,* 67–71.

Segre, L. (2004). Interpersonal psychotherapy for antenatal and postpartum depression. *Primary Psychiatry, 11* (3), 52–56, 66.

Shepard, T.H., Brent, R.L., Friedman, J.M., Jones, K.L., Miller, R.K., Moore, C.A., & Polifka, J.E. (2002). Update on new developments in the study of human teratogens. *Teratology, 65,* 153–161.

Smoller, J.W., & Finn, C.T. (2003). Family, twin, and adoption studies of bipolar disorder. *American Journal of Medical Genetics, 123,* 48–58.

Tennis, P., & Eldridge, R.R. (2002). Preliminary results on pregnancy outcomes in women using lamotrigine. *Epilepsia, 43,* 1161–1167.

Touchette, N., Holtzman, N., Davis, J., & Feetham, S. (1997). *Toward the 21st century: Incorporating genetics into primary health care.* Plainview, New York: Cold Spring Harbor Laboratory Press.

Tsuang, D.W., Faraone, S.V., & Tsuang, M.T. (2001). Genetic counseling for psychiatric disorders. *Current Psychiatric Reports, 3,* 138–143.

Viguera, A.C., Cohen, L.S., Baldessarini, R.J., & Nonacs, R. (2002). Managing bipolar disorder during pregnancy: Weighing the risks and benefits. *Canadian Journal of Psychiatry, 47,* 426–436.

Walker L. (1993). Postpartum depression: One woman's story. *Vancouver Parent, 2,* 14.

Wood, A. F. (1997). The downward spiral of postpartum depression. *American Journal of Maternal/Child Nursing, 6* (22), 308–316.

Yonkers, K.A., Wisner, K.L., Stowe, Z., Leibenluft, E., Cohen, L., & Miller, L. (2004). Management of bipolar disorder during pregnancy and the postpartum period. *American Journal of Psychiatry,* 161, 608–620.

Websites

American Psychiatric Association
www.psych.org

American Psychological Association
www.apa.org

Babycenter
www.babycenter.com

Bipolar Connect
www.bipolarconnect.com

Bipolar Hope
www.bphope.com

Center for Journal Therapy
www.journaltherapy.com

Depression and Bipolar Support Alliance (DBSA)
www.dbsalliance.org

Families for Depression Awareness
www.familyaware.org

March of Dimes
www.marchofdimes.com

Mental Health America
www.mentalhealthamerica.net

National Alliance on Mental Illness (NAMI)
www.nami.org

National Council for Community Behavioral Health Care
www.nccbh.org

National Hopeline Network
www.hopeline.com

National Institute of Mental Health (NIMH)
www.nimh.nih.gov

National Library of Medicine
www.nlm.nih.gov

National Mental Health Information Center (NMHIC)
www.mentalhealth.org

National Strategy for Suicide Prevention
www.mentalhealth.samhsa.gov/suicideprevention

Organization of Teratology Information Specialists (OTIS)
www.otispregnancy.org

Postpartum Dads
www.postpartumdads.org

Postpartum Stress Center
www.postpartumstress.com

Postpartum Support International
www.postpartum.net

Real Savvy Moms
www.realsavvymoms.com

Reprotox
http://reprotox.org
Sleepless in America
www.sleeplessinamerica.org

The Emory Women's Mental Health Program
www.emorywomensprogram.org

TERIS, Teratogen Information System
http://depts.washington.edu/~terisweb/teris

About the Contributors

Jay Carter, PsyD, DABPS, is a licensed psychologist, best-selling author, and professional speaker who conducts seminars and workshops for organizations around the country. He is the author of the bestselling book *Nasty People,* which has sold more than a million copies in the United States and around the world. He is a highly sought-after speaker and has made more than 100 appearances on national television and radio in the United States, Canada, Australia, and Britain (BBC-TV in London). Dr. Carter is a regular speaker on bipolar disorder for Cross Country Education, where his audience comprises social workers, counselors, educators, medical doctors, nurses, nurse practitioners, and psychologists. He has served on the board of directors of the Sexual Assault Resource Center and Women in Crisis (serving battered women) and is past president of the Berks Area Psychological Society.

Ingrid Eerdmans, M.D., is an adult, adolescent, and child psychiatrist, currently practicing in Grand Rapids, Michigan. She has an outpatient practice affiliated with Pine Rest Christian

Mental Health Services that focuses primarily on the treatment of women and children with a broad range of mental disorders. She consults with several residential treatment programs, including Wedgwood Christian Services, that treat severely disordered adolescents. Dr. Eerdmans completed medical school and residency training through Michigan State University's College of Human Medicine. Her twenty-five years in clinical practice have included fourteen years in inpatient and outpatient community mental health settings as well as inpatient and outpatient private practice, mental health administration, and insurance oversight.

Fred Finn, B.S., M.B.A., is the author's husband. The support he has given her throughout the writing of *Bipolar and Pregnant* is invaluable. He was her number one supporter and advocate from preconception through postpartum during both pregnancies; his patience and understanding were pivotal to the success of the births of their daughters. Finn has been employed by the Grand Rapids public schools for twenty years, currently as operations manager of the 21,000-student district. He holds a bachelor's degree in political science from Eastern Michigan University and a master's degree in business administration from Southern Illinois University, and he was an adjunct faculty member at Davenport University in Grand Rapids, Michigan, for five years.

Judith A. Hiemenga, M.D., is an ob-gyn in Grand Rapids, Michigan, in practice at Grand Valley Gynecologists and part of the seven-member Spectrum Health ob-gyn team. Her medical degree is from Michigan State University, and she did her internship and residency at Blodgett, St. Mary's Obstetrics and Gynecology. Dr. Hiemenga is president of the Kent County Medical Society for 2007 and has given television lectures on menopause and osteoporosis. She is the author of the article "On Relationships, Trust and Prevention" in the magazine *Spectrum Health Today.*

Marjorie M. McCulloch, R.N., is the author's mother. A registered nurse for more than forty-five years, she is now semi-retired. She directed a church-sponsored Pregnancy Counseling/ Help Center in Livonia, Michigan, for fifteen years and has been a member of Michigan Nurses for Life, the Genetics Advisory Board of the State of Michigan, and the Perinatal Association of Michigan. Her nursing degree is from Edward W. Sparrow Hospital School of Nursing in Lansing, Michigan. She lives on Suttons Bay in Michigan with her husband, David.

Helga Valdmanis Toriello, Ph.D., a medical geneticist in Grand Rapids, Michigan, is director of Genetics Services at Spectrum Health. She is part of the professional staff at St. Mary's Hospital and Blodgett Memorial Medical Center in Grand Rapids, at Bronson Methodist Hospital in Kalamazoo, and at Mecosta General Hospital in Big Rapids. Dr. Toriello is a professor in the Department of Pediatrics and Human Development at Michigan State University. She received a bachelor of science degree in biology from Cornell University, a master of science degree in genetic counseling from Rutgers University, and a Ph.D. in genetics from Michigan State University. She serves on the Michigan Genetic Advisory Committee as well as on the editorial board of the *Journal of Medical Genetics*.

About the Author

Kristin K. Finn was inspired to write her first book after searching for practical information and guidance on managing her disorder through her pregnancy—from preconception through postpartum—and failed to find resources. Fortunately, she kept a detailed journal, and is able to share her insights written from the unique perspective of someone who lives with a medical illness, particularly bipolar disorder.

Kristin was diagnosed with bipolar disorder when she was nearly seventeen after experiencing turbulent and frightening years, which began in her early teens. After graduating *cum laude* from Western Michigan University, she worked in sales for Xerox Corporation and then for a major pharmaceutical company. Currently Kristin is a successful investment advisor and is an advocate for those affected by bipolar disorder. She is an active member of the Depression and Bipolar Support Alliance (DBSA) Speakers Bureau. She passionately believes that she has a manageable and treatable illness, and her goal is to reduce the social stigma of "mental illness." Kristin enjoys a happy marriage and two beautiful daughters.

Index